Management of Bone Disease and Kidney Failure in Multiple Myeloma

Elena Zamagni
Editor

Management of Bone Disease and Kidney Failure in Multiple Myeloma

A Pocket Guide

Springer

Editor
Elena Zamagni
"Seràgnoli" Institute of Hematology
IRCCS, Azienda Ospedaliera-Universitaria di Bologna
Bologna, Italy

ISBN 978-3-030-63661-6 ISBN 978-3-030-63662-3 (eBook)
https://doi.org/10.1007/978-3-030-63662-3

This Springer imprint is published by the registered company Springer Nature Switzerland AG
The registered company address is: Gewerbestrasse 11, 6330 Cham, Switzerland

Preface

Multiple myeloma is the second most frequent hematologic cancer. According to the pathophysiology of the disease, the clinical picture is mainly characterized by bone involvement and various grades of kidney failure, which are impairing patients' quality of life. Therefore, a correct management of these two important complications is essential for helping patients to face their hopefully long disease course and ultimately for improving the outcomes. Moreover, the cooperation between different specialists is likewise highly important to optimize available resources and all the possible interventions. For this reason, I thought to involve international experts in different fields to finalize this book, which I hope will help oncologists and hematologists in taking care of multiple myeloma patients. I thank all of them for the outstanding contribution.

Bologna, Italy   Elena Zamagni

Contents

Contributors

Rebecca E. Andrews, MRCP, MBChB, BMedSci(hons) Department of Oncology and Metabolism, University of Sheffield, Sheffield, UK

Royal Hallamshire Hospital, Sheffield Teaching Hospitals, Sheffield, UK

A. John Ashcroft, MD Mid Yorkshire NHS Trust, Wakefiled, UK

University of Leeds, Leeds, UK

Clément Bailly, MD Nuclear Medicine Unit, University Hospital, Nantes, France

CRCINA, INSERM, CNRS, Angers University, Nantes University, Nantes, France

Caroline Bodet-Milin, MD Nuclear Medicine Unit, University Hospital, Nantes, France

CRCINA, INSERM, CNRS, Angers University, Nantes University, Nantes, France

Thomas Carlier, MD Nuclear Medicine Unit, University Hospital, Nantes, France

CRCINA, INSERM, CNRS, Angers University, Nantes University, Nantes, France

Andrew D. Chantry, BA, MBChB, MRCP, FRCPath, PhD Department of Oncology and Metabolism, University of Sheffield, Sheffield, UK

Royal Hallamshire Hospital, Sheffield Teaching Hospitals, Sheffield, UK

Claudia Bini, MD Department of Experimental Diagnostic and Specialty Medicine (DIMES), Nephrology, Dialysis and Renal Transplant Unit, S. Orsola-Malpighi Hospital, University of Bologna, Bologna, Italy

Mark A. Cook, PhD Centre for Clinical Haematology, Queen Elizabeth Hospital Birmingham and Institute of Cancer and Genomic Sciences, University of Birmingham, Birmingham, UK

Federica Costa, MD Department of Medicine and Surgery, University of Parma, Parma, Italy

Gillian L. Cribb, MD Montgomery Unit, The Robert Jones and Agnes Hunt Orthopaedic Hospital NHS Foundation Trust, Oswestry, UK

Stefan Delorme, PhD Department of Radiology, German Cancer Research Center, Heidelberg, Germany

Giorgia Comai, MD Department of Experimental Diagnostic and Specialty Medicine (DIMES), Nephrology, Dialysis and Renal Transplant Unit, S. Orsola-Malpighi Hospital, University of Bologna, Bologna, Italy

Nicola Giuliani, PhD Department of Medicine and Surgery, University of Parma, Parma, Italy

Hematology, "Azienda Ospedaliero-Universitaria di Parma", Parma, Italy

Anke Heidemeier, MD Department of Radiology, University Hospital of Würzburg, Würzburg, Germany

Bastien Jamet, MD Nuclear Medicine Unit, University Hospital, Nantes, France

Françoise Kraeber-Bodéré, PhD Nuclear Medicine Unit, University Hospital, Nantes, France

CRCINA, INSERM, CNRS, Angers University, Nantes University, Nantes, France

Nuclear Medicine Unit, ICO-Gauducheau, Nantes-Saint-Herblain, France

Gaetano La Manna, MD, PhD Department of Experimental Diagnostic and Specialty Medicine (DIMES), Nephrology, Dialysis and Renal Transplant Unit, S. Orsola-Malpighi Hospital, University of Bologna, Bologna, Italy

Valentina Marchica, MD Department of Medicine and Surgery, University of Parma, Parma, Italy

Anne-Victoire Michaud, MD Nuclear Medicine Unit, University Hospital, Nantes, France

Philippe Moreau, PhD CRCINA, INSERM, CNRS, Angers University, Nantes University, Nantes, France

Haematology Department, University Hospital, Nantes, France

Cristina Nanni, MD Nuclear Medicine, AOU S.Orsola-Malpighi, Bologna, Italy

Ioannis Ntanasis-Stathopoulos, MD, MSc, PhD Department of Clinical Therapeutics, Alexandra General Hospital, Medical School, National and Kapodistrian University of Athens, Athens, Greece

Leo Rasche, MD Department of Internal Medicine 2, University Hospital of Würzburg, Würzburg, Germany

Mildred Scheel Early Career Center (MSNZ), University Hospital of Würzburg, Würzburg, Germany

Myeloma Center, University of Arkansas for Medical Sciences, Little Rock, AR, USA

Karen L. Shepherd, FRCSEd, MBChB, PhD, BSc (Hons) Montgomery Unit, The Robert Jones and Agnes Hunt Orthopaedic Hospital NHS Foundation Trust, Oswestry, UK

Evangelos Terpos, MD, PhD Department of Clinical Therapeutics, Alexandra General Hospital, Medical School, National and Kapodistrian University of Athens, Athens, Greece

Cyrille Touzeau, MD CRCINA, INSERM, CNRS, Angers University, Nantes University, Nantes, France

Haematology Department, University Hospital, Nantes, France

Valeria Corradetti, MD, PhD Department of Experimental Diagnostic and Specialty Medicine (DIMES), Nephrology, Dialysis and Renal Transplant Unit, S. Orsola-Malpighi Hospital, University of Bologna, Bologna, Italy

Niels Weinhold, MD Myeloma Center, University of Arkansas for Medical Sciences, Little Rock, AR, USA

Department of Internal Medicine V, University Hospital of Heidelberg, Heidelberg, Germany

Elena Zamagni, PhD "Seràgnoli" Institute of Hematology, IRCCS, Azienda Ospedaliera-Universitaria di Bologna, Bologna, Italy

Chapter 1
Introduction: Management of Bone Disease and Kidney Failure in Multiple Myeloma

Elena Zamagni

Multiple myeloma (MM) is a neoplastic disease characterized by proliferation and accumulation of B-lymphocytes and plasma cells (PCs), synthesizing monoclonal immunoglobulin (M component, MC) in the bone marrow (BM) or, more rarely, in extramedullary tissues [1]. The target of the neoplastic transformation is likely a B-lineage cell, and the presence in peripheral blood of B-lymphocytes clonally related to the transformed PCs strongly suggests that the two types of cells might have a common origin. They both derive, during antigen-dependent maturation, in the follicular germi-

E. Zamagni (✉)
"Seràgnoli" Institute of Hematology, IRCCS, Azienda Ospedaliera-Universitaria di Bologna, Bologna, Italy
e-mail: e.zamagni@unibo.it

E. Zamagni (ed.), *Management of Bone Disease and Kidney Failure in Multiple Myeloma*,
https://doi.org/10.1007/978-3-030-63662-3_1

native center, which takes place in secondary lymphoid organs (lymph nodes). Indeed, a common immunoglobulin gene somatic hyper-mutation pattern can be observed in the two types of cells. Neoplastic B-lymphocytes migrate from lymphonodes to BM, where they directly interact with both stromal cells and extracellular matrix. The presence of adhesion molecules on B-lymphocytes surface enhances the interaction with receptors on stromal cells, thus exposing them to cytokines, released from both stromal cells and extracellular matrix. The most crucial cytokine involved in MM growth – both in vivo and in vitro – is IL-6. It exerts both a proliferative and an anti-apoptotic activity and activates osteoclastogenesis. IL-6 production by BM stromal cells is increased as a consequence of the direct contact with PCs, which, in turn, are stimulated by stromal cells to produce other cytokines such as IL-1, TNF-alpha, and M-CSF. These cytokine signals activate stromal cells, other accessory cells, and osteoclasts. Neoplastic PCs stimulate BM angiogenesis as well, throughout the production of VEGF (vascular endothelial growth factor) and FGF (fibroblast growth factor). Increased angiogenesis characterizes the more advanced disease stages. Final disease stages are also characterized by the appearance of a small fraction of highly proliferative plasmoblasts, possibly causing the extramedullary dissemination.

The frequency of MM increases with age and reaches a peak in the 6th–7th life decades. The median age of the population affected is about 65 years old, and less than 10% of all patients come to the diagnosis between the second and fourth decades of life. Males are affected twice as often as females and blacks twice as often compared to the white. The incidence in the latter population is higher than that observed among Asians who live in the same geographic areas. Both genetic and environmental factors are hypothesized to explain racial differences in the incidence of the disease. The main known risk factors are occupational exposure to pesticides, petroleum, and ionizing radiation.

Clinical signs and symptoms at the onset of MM are varied and typically related to the expansion of the neoplastic mass and/or the production by neoplastic cells of cytokines or other factors and/or the peculiar chemical-physical characteristics of the MC [2]. The two most important symptoms, for frequency and severity, are skeletal involvement and renal failure. For this reason, we thought about dedicating a specific book on the management of these two aspects of the disease.

Bone disease is the most frequent feature of MM, occurring in approximately two-thirds of patients at diagnosis and in nearly all patients during their disease [3]. Despite remarkable advances in MM therapy over the last decade, the consequences of skeletal involvement still remain clinically relevant. Bone disease impairs patients' quality of life and represents a major cause of morbidity and mortality. The pathogenesis of skeletal involvement in MM depends on uncoupling of bone remodeling, with increased osteoclast activity, which is unbalanced by adequate osteoblast function. Chapters 2 and 3 will be specifically dedicated to the pathophysiology of bone damage in MM.

The most commonly affected sites are those rich in BM, including the spine, ribs, pelvis, skull, and long bones. Radiologically, the classical aspect of osteolysis is that of a round lesion with sharp margins, well-defined, in the absence of surrounding signs of new bone formation and/or periosteal reaction. In the vertebrae, one can often find crushing aspects and wedging of the body (vertebral fractures). Imaging plays a very important role in the management of MM [4]. First of all, it is necessary for detection of lytic bone lesions, which represent a marker of disease-related end-organ damage, traditionally used to diagnose MM and to establish the need to immediate start of therapy. Additionally, imaging could identify sites of extramedullary disease, which represents an unfavorable prognostic feature and helps to accurately differentiate between solitary plasmacytoma and MM, as well as to predict the risk of early progression from smoldering MM to active disease. During the course of MM, imaging is also essential to establish the diagnosis of relapse and eventually to detect sites of bone damage at potential risk of pathological fractures or neurological complications. Lastly, functional imaging techniques enable more careful assessment of the depth of response to treatment, in particular in patients with non-secretory MM and normal serum free light chain ratio, and more generally contribute to the definition of negative minimal residual disease [5]. Although conventional radiography has traditionally been the standard imaging modality, its low sensitivity in detecting osteolytic lesions and inability to evaluate response to therapy has called for the use of more sophisticated techniques, such as whole-body low-dose computed tomography (WBLDCT), whole-body magnetic resonance imaging (WBMRI), and ^{18}F-fluorodeoxyglucose-positron emission tomography/computed tomography (FDG-PET/CT). Chapters 4, 5, and 6 will be dedicated to imaging techniques in MM, in early phases and for staging, for response assessment and follow-up, with a particular attention to novel imaging techniques.

Agents counteracting bone damage in MM are currently available, namely, antiresorptive agents and drugs targeting bone formation; Chap. 7 will discuss the treatment of bone disease. Orthopedic surgery plays a role as well, which will be discussed in Chap. 8.

Renal impairment is the second most common and most severe complication of MM [6]. It presents in approximately 20% of patients at the time of diagnosis, while another 20–30% of patients develop renal impairment during the course of their disease. The presentation is similar to chronic renal failure, but occasionally patients present with acute failure. The pathogenesis of renal failure in MM is multifactorial. First, and most importantly, it is due to urinary excretion of monoclonal light chains (Bence Jones proteinuria) produced by the neoplastic clone that causes damage to tubules and/or glomeruli by several different mechanisms; this will be the topic of Chap. 9. In addition to urinary excretion of monoclonal light chains, other factors that can contribute to the worsening of renal injury, especially at the onset of the disease, include hypercalcemia, dehydration, use of nephrotoxic drugs (first of all nonsteroidal anti-inflammatory drugs), infections, and hyperuricemia.

Although modern treatment strategies have significantly improved the prognosis of patients with renal failure, the presence of this complication, especially if acute, increases the risk of early mortality within 60 days of MM diagnosis [7]. Many of the novel agents demonstrated to be not only feasible in patients with kidney injury but also to offer the possibility to improve renal function. The treatment of MM with kidney involvement is the topic of Chap. 10.

At the end of this book, the reader will be aware of the physiopathology, clinical presentation, and treatment of the two most important clinical features of MM.

References

1. Kyle RA, Rajkumar SV. Multiple myeloma. N Engl J Med. 2004;351:1860–73.
2. Rajkumar SV, Dimopoulos MA, Palumbo A, et al. International Myeloma Working Group updated criteria for the diagnosis of multiple myeloma. Lancet Oncol. 2014;15:e538–48.
3. Terpos E, Kleber M, Engelhardt M, et al. European Myeloma Network guidelines for the management of multiple myeloma-related complications. Haematologica. 2015;100:1254–66.
4. Zamagni E, Cavo M. The role of imaging techniques in the management of multiple myeloma. Br J Haematol. 2012;159:499–513.
5. Kumar S, Paiva B, Anderson KC, et al. International Myeloma Working Group consensus criteria for response and minimal residual disease assessment in multiple myeloma. Lancet Oncol. 2016;17(8):e328–46.
6. Dimopoulos MA, Terpos E, Chanan-Khan A, et al. Renal impairment in patients with multiple myeloma: a consensus statement on behalf of the International Myeloma Working Group. J Clin Oncol. 2010;28(33):4976–84.
7. Dimopoulos MA, Roussou M, Gkotzamanidou M. The role of novel agents on the reversibility of renal impairment in newly diagnosed symptomatic patients with multiple myeloma. Leukemia. 2013;27(2):423–9.

Chapter 2
The Pathophysiology of Myeloma Bone Disease: Bone Remodelling and the Role of Osteoclasts

Rebecca E. Andrews, Andrew D. Chantry, and A. John Ashcroft

Abbreviations

ALP	Alkaline phosphatase
BAFF	B-cell-activating factor
bALP	Bone alkaline phosphatase
BM	Bone marrow

The original version of this chapter was revised. The correction to this chapter can be found at https://doi.org/10.1007/978-3-030-63662-3_11

R. E. Andrews · A. D. Chantry
Department of Oncology and Metabolism, University of Sheffield, Sheffield, UK

Royal Hallamshire Hospital, Sheffield Teaching Hospitals, Sheffield, UK

A. J. Ashcroft (✉)
Mid Yorkshire NHS Trust, Wakefiled, UK

University of Leeds, Leeds, UK
e-mail: aj.ashcroft@nhs.net

E. Zamagni (ed.), *Management of Bone Disease and Kidney Failure in Multiple Myeloma*,
https://doi.org/10.1007/978-3-030-63662-3_2

BMD	Bone mineral density
BMME	Bone marrow microenvironment
BMP-2	Bone morphogenetic protein-2
BMSC	Bone marrow stromal cells
CBFA1	Core-binding factor Runt domain α subunit 1
CCL3	Chemokine (C-C motif) ligand 3
DcR3	Decoy receptor 3
DKK1	Dickopf-1
FRP	Frizzled-related proteins
Gfi1	Growth factor independence 1
HGF	Hepatocyte growth factor
IL-	Interleukin-
LRP	Low-density lipoprotein receptor-related protein
MBD	Myeloma bone disease
MGUS	Monoclonal gammopathy of unknown significance
MIP	Macrophage inflammatory protein
MM	Multiple myeloma
MMP	Matrix metalloproteinase
MPC	Malignant plasma cell
NF κB	Nuclear factor kappa B
OAFs	Osteoclast-activating factors
OB	Osteoblast
OC	Osteoclast
OIFs	Osteoblast-inhibiting factors
OP	Osteoporosis
OPG	Osteoprotegerin
PTH	Parathyroid hormone
PTHrP	Parathyroid hormone-related protein
RANK	Receptor activator of nuclear factor kappa B
RANKL	Receptor activator of nuclear factor kappa B ligand
Runx2	Runt-related transcription factor 2
SDF-1 α	Stromal cell-derived factor 1 α (also known as CXCL12)
sFRP-	Secreted frizzled-related protein-
SRE	Skeletal-related events
TGF-β	Transforming growth factor-beta
TNF	Tumour necrosis factor
TRAF6	TNF receptor-associated factor 6

TRAIL	TNF-related apoptosis-inducing ligand
VCAM1	Vascular cell adhesion molecule-1
VLA4	Very late antigen 4 (also known as α4β1 integrin)
WIF-1	Wnt inhibitory factor 1
Wnt	Wingless/Intergrase-1

Introduction

Myeloma-induced bone disease (MBD) is thought to affect 80–90% of patients with myeloma [1, 2] at some point during their disease journey. The associated loss of trabecular bone, reduced bone mineral density (BMD) and osteolytic lesions leads to significant disease burden and subsequent impact on patient quality of life. Sufferers experience bone pain, decreased mobility and, in severe cases, spinal cord compression-induced paralysis. Patients with a diagnosis of myeloma are nine times more likely to develop a skeletal-related event (SRE) [3], and those who experience a pathological fracture have over 20% increased mortality [4]. The importance of understanding this clinical phenomenon and managing the impact of this disease on patients remains paramount. In view of the complexities of the bone marrow microenvironment, the intricacies of MBD pathophysiology continue to be explored. Here we review the specific role of the osteoclast in this devastating pathological process, after first addressing an overview of the basics of normal bone physiology. The roles of both the osteoblast and osteocyte will be discussed in a later chapter.

Normal Physiology of Bone

Anatomy of Bone

The human skeleton allows engineered multifunctionality: structure, motility and protection of internal organs, as well having a crucial role in calcium metabolism and haematopoiesis. There are 206 individual bones within the mature axial and appendicular human skeleton combined. Bones vary in shape and structure and can be subcategorised into long, short, flat or irregular (including sesamoid) bones. Differing ratios of cortical vs. trabecular bone mass influence bone characteristics and properties. Cortical bone is thought to account for approximately 80% of total bone volume in the human skeleton and has higher mineral content in comparison to trabecular bone and thus higher biomechanical resistance. Trabecular bone forms a porous honeycomb-type structure, comprising rods and plates, giving strength which is stress adaptive with comparatively lower bone mass. Long bones, such as the femur (the largest human bone), generally have a thick cortex for mechanical resistance in skeletal locomotion. In contrast, the stapes bone (the smallest bone in the human body) is an intricate and uniquely shaped bone with site-specific qualities to allow conduction of sound waves. The remarkable design and adaptability of healthy human bone are made possible by the complex bone marrow microenvironment, consisting of both a cellular and non-cellular (or extracellular) compartment, which will be discussed in more detail below.

Extracellular Matrix

Overall bone composition is approximately 50–70% mineral, 20–40% protein/organic matrix and 5–10% water [5]. The extracellular matrix protein composition is mainly collagenous (up to 85–90%), with type I collagen the most abundant. Collagen fibres are mineralised by calcium hydroxyapatite ($Ca_5(PO_4)_3OH$), increasing biomechanical strength of the underlying matrix. Other non-collagenous aspects of the matrix consist of proteins such as proteoglycans, glycosylated proteins and gamma-carboxylated (gla) proteins [5]. These proteins help facilitate bone remodelling and mineralisation. These are via cellular pathways particularly, but not exclusively, involving cells specific to the bone marrow environment: osteoblasts (OBs), osteoclasts (OCs) and osteocytes. Active vitamin D (1,25-$(OH)_2$D) supports mineralisation by promoting absorption of calcium and phosphate from the gut, as well as promoting differentiation of OBs that ultimately facilitate mineralisation. The collagenous matrix allows for bone flexibility, whereas mineralisation leads to bone strength and rigidity, with both characteristics required for optimal bone functionality.

Bone Cells

Osteoclasts

Osteoclasts (OCs) originate from hematopoietic cells and differentiate via the monocyte/macrophage lineage into multinucleated cells. Commitment to this differentiation is achieved in the presence of macrophage colony-stimulating factor (M-CSF) and receptor activator of nuclear factor kappa B ligand (RANKL) (Fig. 2.1). M-CSF and RANKL are both expressed by osteoblasts and bone marrow stromal cells, promoting differentiation and survival of OC precursor cells. M-CSF allows for early OC differentiation. RANKL binding with receptor activator of nuclear factor kappa B (RANK) expressed on the OC cell surface leads to mature OC differentiation via TNF receptor-associated factor 6 (TRAF6) and nuclear factor kappa B (NF κB) [6]. Osteoprotegerin (OPG), the soluble decoy receptor to RANKL, is produced by osteoblasts, to regulate appropriate OC proliferation and activity (Fig. 2.3).

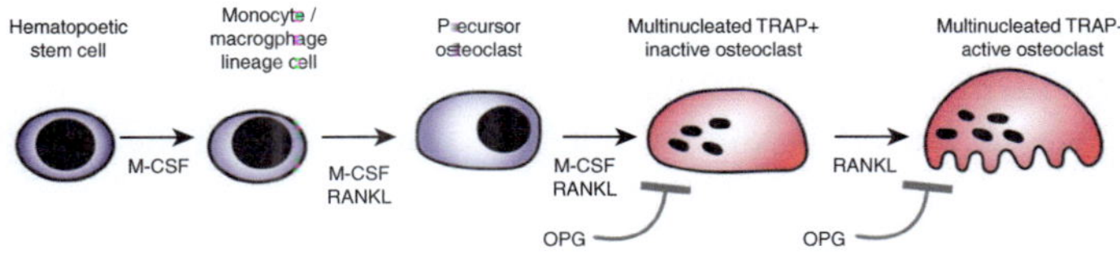

FIGURE 2.1 Osteoclastogenesis. Osteoclasts are derived from hematopoietic stem cells. In the presence of factors such as macrophage colony-stimulating factor (M-CSF) and receptor activator of nuclear factor kappa B ligand (RANKL), precursor OC cells differentiate into multinucleated osteoclast cells, which when activated are capable of bone resorption. Osteoclastogenesis can be inhibited by the production of OPG, which can bind to RANKL, preventing it binding to RANK on the OC cell surface

Hence, the balance of RANKL/OPG can either lead to increased or decreased bone resorption in response to physiological stimuli and/or pathological states.

OCs account for approximately 2% of the total number of bone cells within the adult BMME, unless there is a pre-existing pathology that alters these numbers. OCs are defined as cells that have at least three nuclei and have the ability to resorb bone. Resorption is made possible in part because of the unique ruffled border structure of the OC, which allows cells to attach and create a seal on the bone surface. Once a seal has been made, OCs release H^+-ATPase which causes a release of protons to induce an acidic environment, as well as releasing proteolytic enzymes (e.g. cathepsin K) and matrix metalloproteinase (MMP) [7]. The acidic conditions lead to demineralisation of the matrix, and, subsequently, the enzymes released break down the exposed collagen fibres.

Osteoblasts

Osteoblasts (OBs) account for approximately 5% of total bone cells in the adult bone marrow microenvironment (BMME) and are the only cells known to be responsible for forming a new bone. OBs are mesenchymal stem cell-derived mononuclear cells that differentiate in the presence of transcription factors such as β-catenin, Runt-related transcription factor 2 (Runx2) and Osterix (Fig. 2.2).

Wingless/Intergrase-1 (Wnt) signalling is the predominant regulator of OB proliferation, differentiation and activity, driving lineage via a number of pathways. One such pathway is via increased β-catenin via the canonical Wnt signalling pathway, which increases Runx2 promotion of osteoblastogenesis. Alternative signalling is via expression of transforming growth factor-beta (TGF-β) and bone morphogenetic protein-2 (BMP-2), which both support OB differentiation via Smad/Runx2. Runx2 can also drive RANKL/OPG expression to regulate cell differentiation. In addition to this, anti-apoptotic cell conditions are facilitated via Src/ERK and PI3K/AKT proteins [8], again via Wnt signalling. Wnt/Ca2+

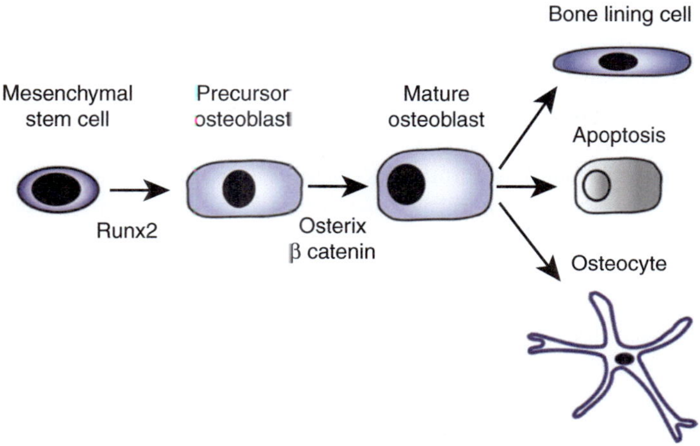

FIGURE 2.2 Osteoblast differentiation. Osteoblasts are derived from mesenchymal stem cells. Commitment to the osteoblast lineage is regulated by multiple pathways, of which the more established involve Wnt signalling cascades. Mature osteoblasts subsequently either apoptose, become entrapped within the bone matrix to form osteocytes or differentiate into bone-lining cells

(the non-canonical Wnt signalling) also supports OB differentiation via upregulation of Osterix. There are multiple inhibitors of the Wnt pathway, such as DKK1 and sFRP1. Following active bone formation, OBs either apoptose, differentiate into osteocytes (within the bone matrix) or differentiate into bone-lining cells that protect the bone throughout quiescence.

Osteocytes

Osteocyte cells are derived from mature OBs, when an OB becomes surrounded by mineralised bone matrix. They account for approximately 90–95% of the bone cells found in healthy adult bone [9]. Within the last 10 years, there has been increasing interest in osteocytes, in particular their role in the communication between cells within the BMME and regulation of bone turnover. Wnt/β-catenin is as important to osteocytes as it appears to be for OBs. Unlike OBs that use this signalling to proliferate, differentiate and form bone matrix, osteocytes appear to use Wnt/β-catenin signalling in response to mechanical loading. Mechanical loading appears to decrease the release of sclerostin and Dkk-1 (inhibitors of Wnt signalling) from osteocytes, therefore promoting this Wnt/β-catenin signalling pathway and increasing bone formation. Osteocytes have been demonstrated in vivo to be a major source of RANKL production and therefore also play a crucial role in OC activity [10].

Osteocytes are increasingly being recognised as the master regulators of bone remodelling, carefully orchestrating the drive of either bone formation or resorption in response to environmental factors (such as biomechanical loading). They remain notoriously difficult to research in vitro, due to the technical difficulty of isolating osteocytes from a calcified bone matrix and then maintaining their phenotype within a representative culture environment to allow for experimentation [11].

Physiological Bone Remodelling

In early adult life, the shape of bone adapts within the skeleton by adding or removing bone in the process of bone modelling. Once matured, skeletal health is maintained by the process of bone remodelling (Fig. 2.3), the regulated balance of bone resorption (removal) by osteoclast cells and bone formation by osteoblast cells. The remodelling of bone is a cyclical process, initiated in response to physiological mechanical loading or microfracture damage to the bone. It is thought that osteocyte cells respond to biomechanical stimuli or damage and orchestrate cellular interactions that lead to OC precursor recruitment to required areas of the bone matrix. One such pathway is via bone-lining cells, which are activated by factors released from the bone matrix (e.g. interleukin-6 (IL-6)), leading to RANKL surface expression, which subsequently attracts OC precursor cells [12]. This is

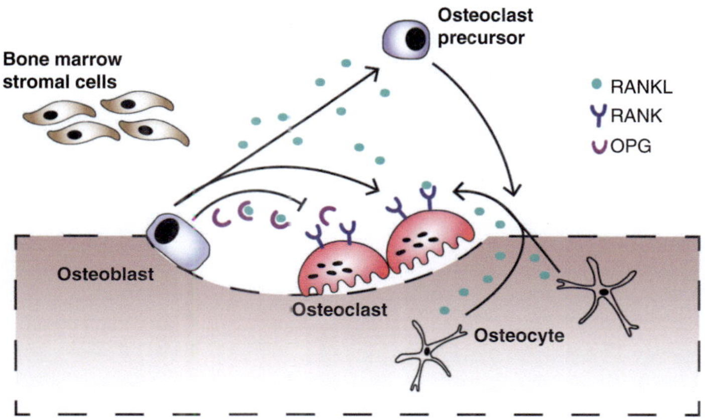

FIGURE 2.3 RANKL/RANK/OPG interaction. There is a close relationship between RANKL and OPG to either drive or antagonise OC differentiation, function and survival. RANKL is produced by both osteocytes and osteoblasts, and when bound to RANK on the surface of osteoclast precursors and immature osteoclasts, differentiation and maturation take place. This signalling pathway is moderated by osteoprotegerin (OPG), a decoy receptor to RANKL which is expressed by osteoblasts, to downregulate OC formation

known as the activation phase, which is followed by a phase of resorption. Of particular importance in this phase is the ratio of RANKL to OPG (higher RANKL to OPG increases bone resorption), as well as other cytokines such as interleukin-1 (IL-1), IL-6 and parathyroid hormone (PTH) to name a few. A reversal phase follows resorption and is the point when resorption is complete. Growth factors released from the bone matrix during resorption will have signalled OB precursor recruitment in preparation for bone formation in the resorption pit. During the formation phase, new unmineralised matrix osteoid is produced, which will later be mineralised, producing strong healthy new bone. Osteoblasts that do not apoptose differentiate into either osteocytes (if incorporated into the bone matrix) or bone-lining cells. At this stage, remodelling is complete and the bone enters a quiescent phase (Fig. 2.4).

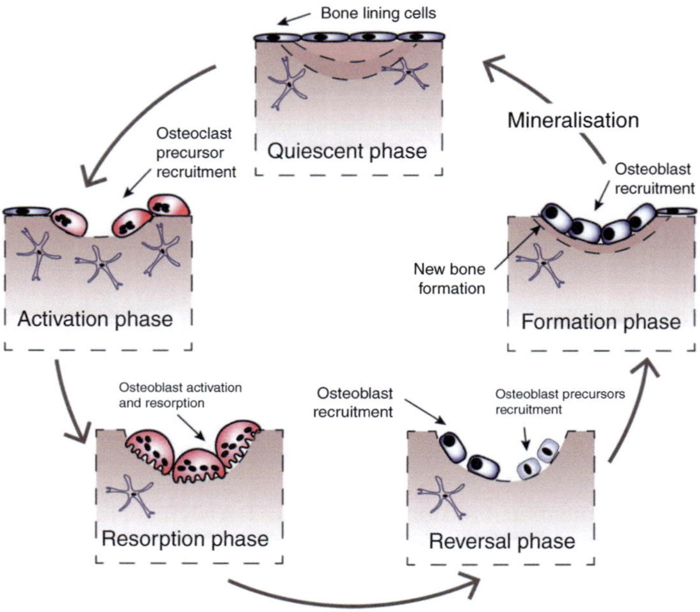

FIGURE 2.4 Physiological bone remodelling. Bone remodelling involves five distinct phases. Initially, bone microdamage or mechanical loading is recognised by osteocyte cells. Osteocyte-mediated intracellular signalling then triggers an activation phase in which osteoclast precursor cells are recruited to the area of the bone. Subsequent osteoclast maturation, recruitment and bone resorption follow. It is not understood what leads to the transition from resorption to formation, but in this so-called reversal phase, the osteoclasts' role is complete, and osteoblast precursors are recruited. The final active phase is that of bone formation. Osteoblasts lay down osteoid (a new collagen matrix) which will be later mineralised. On completion of the cycle, osteoblast cells either apoptose, become engulfed in the matrix and become osteocytes, or differentiate into bone lining cells that protect the surface of the new bone

It is thought that approximately 10% of the adult human skeleton is replaced each year via this remodelling process. This maintenance and repair optimise bone health and strength, as well as playing a crucial role in ongoing calcium homeostasis. Bone remodelling rates change throughout life, with a significant accrual of bone mass seen throughout childhood/adolescent years, followed by a relatively stable period of bone turnover during adult life. Optimal bone mass is usually reached by aged 30 [13]. In later life, there is a gradual reduction in bone mass, observed in both men and women, with many suffering with osteoporosis requiring bone strengthening pharmacological intervention. Osteoporosis is defined by the World Health Organisation as a BMD equal to or less than 2.5 standard deviations below that of the average reference BMD of a young (20–29 years old) female [14]. The aging skeleton is particularly associated with changes in oestrogen levels, and hence post-menopausal women are particularly susceptible to more rapid reductions in BMD in comparison to age-matched men.

This constant remodelling process maintains bone shape and strength. During early life, human bone undergoes growth from growth plates, as well as bone modelling, a process by which biomechanical forces change the shape of the bone as an adaption to environmental alterations. Unlike remodelling, these processes are more frequently required in the immature skeleton or pathological states.

The Pathophysiology of Myeloma Bone Disease

In myeloma, interaction between bone marrow stromal cells and MPCs leads to dysregulation of bone remodelling. One of the key foundations of MBD pathophysiology is that of the initial adherence of MPCs to stromal cells in the BMME. Adhesion molecules such as vascular cell adhesion molecule-1 (VCAM1) and very late antigen 4 (VLA4, also known as α4β1 integrin) promote MPC proliferation and habitability within the BMME, as well as concurrently catalysing alterations in the bone remodelling cycle [15]. The notch signalling pathways are also of importance in MPC adhesion to stromal cells, with MPCs releasing Notch (Notch 1, 2 and 3), which interacts with Jagged to result in upregulation of RANKL (increasing osteoclastogenesis) [16, 17]. Syndecan-1, expressed on the surface of MPCs, also assists adhesion and subsequently supports tumour growth (via HGF and cMet), as well as affecting bone turnover [18].

Dysregulation of bone remodelling can be via direct cellular interactions or release of cytokines or extracellular vesicles. Factors influencing alterations in the equilibrium of bone remodelling are often categorised as osteoclast-activating factors (OAFs) and osteoblast-inhibiting factors (OIFs). Myeloma plasma cells (MPCs) produce these factors to directly exhibit changes to OB and OC function, as well as indirectly orchestrating intracellular signalling within the BMME. Subsequent uncoupling of OB and OC activity results in upregulated osteoclastic activity and downregulated osteoblastic activity, leading to net loss of bone. Bone undergoes pathological changes resulting in trabecular bone loss, with or without defined osteolytic lesions [19]. Dysregulated molecular cascades and cellular pathways are identified in MM, some of which are of importance in the development of the oncolytic bone phenotype [20].

The increased resorption demonstrated in MBD subsequently enhances the release of additional chemokines, cytokines and growth factors from the bone matrix. These further drive OC and OB dysregulation, as well as positively supporting MPCs proliferation and encouraging further neoplastic homing to the BMME. It is for this reason that MBD is often described as a "vicious cycle", as the oncolytic changes in the BMME promote future cancer survival (see Fig. 2.5).

Osteoclast-Activating Factors

Numerous OAFs have been identified, which promote OC differentiation, proliferation, action and/or survival. It is appreciated that MPCs directly produce some of the factors that have been associated with osteoclastogenesis. The most frequently documented include IL-3, TNFα, macrophage

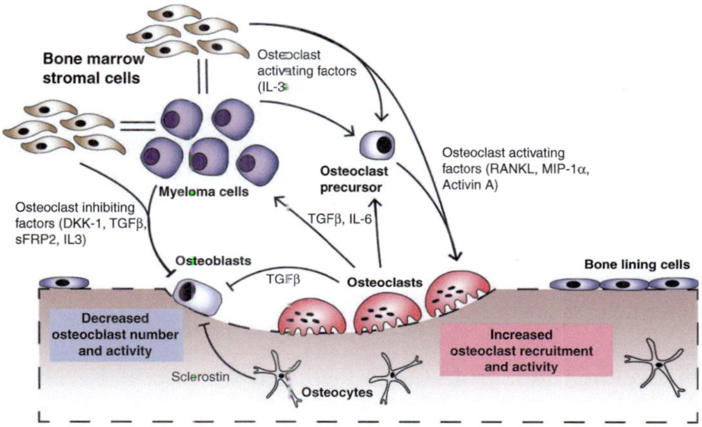

FIGURE 2.5 Myeloma bone disease: a vicious cycle. The pathophysiology of myeloma bone disease: Cellular interaction between myeloma plasma cells (MPCs) and bone marrow stromal cells (BMSCs) leads to factors that influence the equilibrium of bone turnover. Osteoclast-activating factors (e.g. IL-3, RANKL, MIP-1α and activin A) are released both from myeloma cells directly and indirect upregulation as a result of adhesion between MPCs and BMSCs. Increased resorption results in increased release of factors such as TGFβ and IL-6 from the bone marrow matrix. These promote a positive feedback with upregulation of MPC and osteoclast precursor proliferation, as well as inhibiting osteoblastogenesis. Osteoblast-inhibiting factors (e.g. DKK-1, TGFβ, sFRP2, IL-3) are also released as a result of the presence of MPCs and their interaction with BMSCs. These factors antagonise osteoblast differentiation and function. Sclerostin released from osteocytes is also upregulated in the presence of MPCs, which also inhibits osteoblast function. The overall effect of this is an increase in osteoclast activity and decreased osteoblast activity, resulting in osteolytic bone disease

inflammatory protein-1 α (MIP-1α), MIP-1β and decoy receptor 3 (DcR3). MPCs are also thought to indirectly impact on local bone marrow cell signalling, particularly following adhesion to BMSCs, causing OAFs to be released from the local bone marrow environment (e.g. from bone marrow stromal cells). In addition, osteoclasts also directly release OAFs (including activin A and MIP-1α), self-promoting osteoclast activity. Clinical studies have confirmed that bone resorption markers are not only raised in MM patients but also in MGUS patients that later progress to MM (suggesting potential uses in predicting disease progression) [21]. OAFs are summarised within this section, but those discussed are not exhaustive.

RANKL/RANK/OPG

In myeloma, numerous OAFs facilitate increases in RANKL, the role of which in bone physiology has previously been discussed (Fig. 2.3). OAFs identified to promote RANKL include PTH, parathyroid hormone-related protein (PTHrP), IL-1, IL-7, tumour necrosis factor-α (TNFα) and glucocorticoids [22], some of which are expressed by MPCs directly.

In healthy individuals, RANKL is released by BMSCs, T cells and OBs. RANKL binds to RANK on immature precursor OCs, causing OC differentiation to mature multinucleated cells, capable of regulated bone resorption. In myeloma, OAFs drive upregulation of RANK-RANKL binding, supporting increased OC maturation, and decreased inhibition of OC apoptosis. Physiologically, this would be counterbalanced by OPG, produced by OBs to act as a decoy receptor to RANKL, blocking RANK-RANKL binding. In MBD, however, not only are RANKL levels raised [23, 24], but OPG levels are inappropriately low [25]. This altered RANKL/OPG ratio causes net bone loss and osteolytic bone disease [26]. RANKL is potentially released directly from MPCs [27, 28], but this is not universally supported, with some research groups proposing that increased RANKL is due to increased expression from BMSCs [29].

In vivo MBD models receiving treatment with recombinant OPG had reduced development of osteolytic lesions, demonstrating that RANKL blockage leads to improved disease outcomes [30]. Anti-RANKL monoclonal antibody, Denosumab (XGEVA®, Amgen), was shown in clinical trial to promote anti-catatonic effects, reducing rates of SREs [31]. This treatment is now approved in the context of myeloma and will be discussed in more detail in later chapters.

Both physiological plasma cells and MPCs also express syndecan-1, a transmembrane proteoglycan. Investigators have demonstrated that reduced OPG levels in MM are likely, in part, related to MPC overexpression of syndecan-1, which has the ability to bind and degrade OPG. The resulting unopposed RANK-RANKL binding in this OPG deplete environment is another mechanism driving osteolysis [32]. T cells also promote osteoclastogenesis in MM patients via the release of RANKL, OPG and TNF-related apoptosis-inducing ligand (TRAIL). TRAIL normally supports cell apoptosis, but in the presence of MM cells, OPG and TRAIL form complexes that support OC survival.

Macrophage Inflammatory Protein-1 A (MIP-1A)

MIP-1α (also known as CCL-3) is a CC chemokine shown to be increased in serum and BM clinical samples in patients with MM [24, 33–35], in part due to altered expression of transcription factors from myeloma cells (namely, acute myeloid leukaemia-1A and acute myeloid leukaemia-1B [36]). Released by MPCs and BMSCs, MIP-1α supports later stages of osteoclastogenesis via CCR1- and CCR5-binding receptors on the OC cell surface [26, 37, 38]. Higher MIP-1α levels correlate to more severe MBD [39], as well as higher RANKL levels [34]. Surplus RANKL is released by BMSCs as a result of increased MIP-1 expression. In vivo, MIP-1α enhanced osteoclast differentiation induced by IL-6, RANKL and PTHrP. In addition, antibody blockade of MIP-1α in vitro leads to normalisation of osteoclast formation in myeloma samples [40]. This is further supported by in vivo studies in which blockade of MIP-1α reduced osteoclastogenesis, subsequent MBD, and also reduced tumour homing to the BMME, increasing survival of the malignant clone [37, 41]. MIP-1β (also known as CCL-4) is also expressed by a number of myeloma cell lines and supports preosteoclast lineage to drive osteolysis [33]. Another CC chemokine implicated in MBD is MIP-3α (also known as CCL-20) which is overexpressed by OB and OCs in the presence of MPCs. This overexpression has been shown to drive the differentiation of mature osteoclasts, and blockade of anti-MIP-3α antibody in vitro leads to inhibition of OC formation [42].

Interleukins (IL)

A number of the interleukins are thought to stimulate osteoclastogenesis. IL-6 is mainly produced by BMSCs and is not only implicated in the promotion of MPC proliferation and survival but also enhances osteoclast differentiation [43]. Levels of IL-6 expression are elevated in advanced stages of MM [44] and are thought to induce osteoclastogenesis by promoting RANKL as well as indirectly via other OAFs [45]. Treatment with human anti- IL-6 antibody in a myeloma xenograft model resulted in reduced myeloma tumour burden as well as a reduction in osteolytic disease [46]. Another interleukin thought to be of significance to MBD pathophysiology is IL-3, which has been shown to be expressed by plasma cells isolated from human bone marrow samples from myeloma sufferers. IL-3 appears to be upregulated in the presence of increased transcription factors released from MPCs (including acute myeloid leukaemia-1A and acute myeloid leukaemia 1B). IL-3 stimulates MPC survival, as well as driving early osteoclast differentiation [47]. Both MIP-1α- and RANKL-induced osteoclastogenic effects appear to be enhanced by IL-3 in vitro, suggesting a potential future therapeutic target for treatment of MBD. IL-1β is also elevated in MM, in comparison to controls [48, 49], especially in those with established osteolytic lesions [50]. It is thought that IL-1β may have a role as an OAF by driving increased IL-6 and therefore further resorption activity. IL-17, released by T lymphocytes within the BMME, is also overexpressed due to the release of other cytokines, namely, IL-6, IL-1β and TGFβ. This interleukin has also been demonstrated at increased levels in the BM and correlates to the presence of MBD, thought to be due to upregulation of RANKL-induced osteoclastogenesis [39]. IL-11 also has a potential role in osteoclast formation and is expressed by OB cells. A recent study suggests that IL-11 can be induced by HGF, via a number of pathways including extracellular vesicles [51].

Vascular Endothelial Growth Factor

Vascular endothelial growth factor (VEGF) is a cytokine involved in multiple systemic roles, including angiogenesis, stem cell development and inflammation. Regarding bone, VEGF has been shown to be important in osteoclastogenesis, supposedly as a result of interactions between the BMME, MPCs and vascular endothelial cells [28]. VEGF is released from MPCs, OCs and BMSCs at higher levels than seen in controls [52, 53]. Increases in VEGF have corresponded to increases in other cytokines, IL-6, IL-1β and TNFα, known to be of importance in myeloma cell survival and in driving MBD [54].

Osteopontin

Osteopontin (OPN) is a matrix protein involved in many aspects of human physiology. Levels of OPN are often elevated in MM, with OPN released from MPCs and also expressed at increased levels from BMSCs of MM patients [55]. Increased levels of OPN have been associated with established lytic bone lesions [56]. One role of OPN has been identified as cooperating with VEGF to drive angiogenic changes within the BMME of MM patients [53]. In addition, OPN is thought to be expressed from BMSCs in MM patients, increasing tumour cell migration and adhesion, and therefore promotes further tumour and MBD progression via this vicious cycle [55].

Other Factors

As well as the previously mentioned OAFs, further factors associated with upregulated bone resorption are described, although the roles of some are still under exploration. PTHrP is released by MPCs and MM cell lines [57] and acts via its receptor PTHR1 to promote pro-osteoclastic effects. When investigating PTHrP in the context of myeloma, PTHrP release from MPCs was shown to upregulate RANKL and thus gross bone volume loss [57]; however in vivo studies demonstrated challenges in therapeutic targeting in the context of MBD. SDF-1α, produced by BMSC, is measured at increased levels in patients with myeloma (especially those with bone disease) compared to healthy controls [58]. Its role in the homing and adhesion of MPCs to the BMME has previously been described, with increased chemotherapy resistance demonstrated via IL-6 in vitro [59]. Increasing SDF-1α enhances OC precursor proliferation and differentiation. Soluble decoy receptor-3 (DcR3) is a member of the tumour necrosis factor (TNF) receptor family and is expressed by T lymphocytes and MM cells from myeloma patients [60]. DcR3 has a role in promoting MPC survival, as well as supporting the OC lineage via upregulation of RANKL and TNFα [60]. Another member of the TNF family is B-cell-activating factor (BAFF), which is a cytokine expressed by BMSCs and at increased levels in MM patients [61–63]. BAFF appears to promote osteoclastogenesis independent of RANKL, possibly via MCSF. Transforming growth factor-β (TGF-β) has been predominantly been targeted in the context of MBD for its anti-anabolic effects; however, TGF-β also plays a role in OC formation and function, and in vivo therapies blocking receptor to TGF-β receptor 1 have demonstrated anti-catatonic, as well as anabolic effects [64]. Another factor thought to have both pro-resorptive and anti-anabolic effects is activin A, which is a glycoprotein, detected at higher levels in patient with myeloma [65]. In vitro, activin A enhanced expression of RANK and therefore is thought to support early osteoclastogenesis [66, 67].

Advances in laboratory techniques have increased research understanding into myeloma-derived extracellular vesicles and the proteins and microRNAs that are carried via this intercellular process. The microRNA, miR-21, has been shown to be upregulated clinically. During in vitro co-culture of BMSCs with MPCs, there was a subsequent increased RANKL-OPG expression from BMSCs [68]. This altered RANKL-OPG balance supports osteoclastogenesis and subsequent osteolysis. There are increasing publications in this area, and it is likely that our scientific understanding in this area will rapidly increase in the coming years (Table 2.1).

TABLE 2.1 Osteoclast-activating factors (OAFs) identified as directly or indirectly influencing myeloma bone disease pathophysiology

Factor	**Source**	**Action**	**Reference**
Activin A	OBs	Supports OC precursor lineage, as well as playing a role as an OIF	[35, 66]
BAFF	MPCs and OCs	Promotes MCS-F-induced osteoclastogenesis and MPC survival	[61–63]
DcR3	T cells and MPCs	Increases RANKL and TNFα, increasing osteoclastogenesis	[60, 69]
Dkk-1	MPCs	Predominantly an OIF, but also inhibits Wnt3a-regulated OPG, increasing osteolysis	[35, 70, 71]
HGF	MPCs	Supports osteoclast activation by increasing IL-11	[72–74]
IL-1β	MPCs	Increases OC formation	[75]
IL-3	MPCs	Increases pre-OC numbers and fusion to mature OCs, promotes MM cell growth, and upregulates activin A	[47, 76, 77]
IL-6	BMSCs and OBs	Increases proliferation and survival of OCs and MPCs	[43, 44, 47, 74, 76]
IL-11	OBs	Increases OC recruitment and activation	[51, 73]

Table 2.1 (continued)

Factor	Source	Action	Reference
MIP-1α	MPCs	Increases OC differentiation and recruitment (via CCR1 and CCR5 receptors). Enhances MPC survival and growth	[35, 78]
MIP-1β	MPCs	Increases OC differentiation/ recruitment	[33]
MIP-3α	OBs and OCs	Increases OC differentiation in the presence of IL-1	[35]
miR-21	BMSCs	Alters RANKL-OPG expression, supporting osteoclastogenesis	[68]
Notch	MPCs	Alters Notch-Jagged interactions, increasing osteoclastogenesis	[16, 17]
Osteopontin	OBs, OCs, BMSCs, some MPCs	Supports osteoclast resorption and promotes MPC survival via IL-6	[56, 79]
PTHrP	MPCs	Enhances osteoclastogenesis	[57]
RANKL	BMSCs	Increases osteoclastogenesis and reduces OC apoptosis via RANKL-RANK binding	[28, 80]
SDF-1α	BMSC	Increases MMP-9, increasing osteoclast activation and motility	[58, 81, 82]

(continued)

TABLE 2.1 (continued)

Factor	Source	Action	Reference
Syndecan-1	MPCs	Binds OPG, reducing RANKL inhibition	[32]
TNFα	MPCs	Increases OC differentiation and therefore osteolysis, by increasing RANKL Promotes MM cell growth via IL-6	[19, 83]
TGFβ	OBs	Promotes early OC differentiation	[19, 64]
TRAF6	BMSCs	Binds RANK, causing TRAF6 trimer release and further downstream RANK	[84–86]
VEGF	MPCs and BMME	Supports osteoclastogenesis, also increases IL-6 which increases MP proliferation	[52, 53]
XBP1	BMSC	Increases RANKL, promoting osteoclastogenesis	[87]

Conclusion

The understanding of MBD pathophysiology and the role that osteoclasts play in the complex bone microenvironment continues to be explored and hence remains an exciting and ever-changing research field. It is important to continue to scrutinise our understanding of this devastating phenomenon, in order for researchers to develop improved therapeutic options for patients afflicted. Although there has been good progress in clinical research in the past decade, it is likely that the coming years will bring a vast number of changes both in scientific discovery and in therapeutic options clinically to benefit patient management.

References

1. Kyle RA, Gertz MA, Witzig TE, Lust JA, Lacy MQ, Dispenzieri A, et al. Review of 1027 patients with newly diagnosed multiple myeloma. Mayo Clin Proc. 2003;78(1):21–33.
2. Coleman RE. Skeletal complications of malignancy. Cancer. 1997;80(8 Suppl):1588–94.
3. Melton LJ 3rd, Kyle RA, Achenbach SJ, Oberg AL, Rajkumar SV. Fracture risk with multiple myeloma: a population-based study. J Bone Miner Res. 2005;20(3):487–93.
4. Saad F, Lipton A, Cook R, Chen YM, Smith M, Coleman R. Pathologic fractures correlate with reduced survival in patients with malignant bone disease. Cancer. 2007;110(8):1860–7.
5. Clarke B. Normal bone anatomy and physiology. Clin J Am Soc Nephrol. 2008;3(Suppl 3):S131–9.
6. Kearns AE, Khosla S, Kostenuik PJ. Receptor activator of nuclear factor kappaB ligand and osteoprotegerin regulation of bone remodeling in health and disease. Endocr Rev. 2008;29(2):155–92.
7. Feng X, Teitelbaum SL. Osteoclasts: new insights. Bone Res. 2013;1(1):11–26.
8. Yavropoulou MP, Yovos JG. The role of the Wnt signaling pathway in osteoblast commitment and differentiation. Hormones (Athens). 2007;6(4):279–94.
9. Bonewald LF, Johnson ML. Osteocytes, mechanosensing and Wnt signaling. Bone. 2008;42(4):606–15.
10. Nakashima T, Hayashi M, Fukunaga T, Kurata K, Oh-Hora M, Feng JQ, et al. Evidence for osteocyte regulation of bone homeostasis through RANKL expression. Nat Med. 2011;17(10):1231–4.
11. Shah KM, Stern MM, Stern AR, Pathak JL, Bravenboer N, Bakker AD. Osteocyte isolation and culture methods. Bonekey Rep. 2016;5:838.
12. Rucci N. Molecular biology of bone remodelling. Clin Cases Miner Bone Metab. 2008;5(1):49–56.
13. Henry YM, Fatayerji D, Eastell R. Attainment of peak bone mass at the lumbar spine, femoral neck and radius in men and

women: relative contributions of bone size and volumetric bone mineral density. Osteoporos Int. 2004;15(4):263–73.
14. Kanis JA, McCloskey EV, Johansson H, Oden A, Melton LJ 3rd, Khaltaev N. A reference standard for the description of osteoporosis. Bone. 2008;42(3):467–75.
15. Katz BZ. Adhesion molecules--the lifelines of multiple myeloma cells. Semin Cancer Biol. 2010;20(3):186–95.
16. Terpos E, Ntanasis-Stathopoulos I, Gavriatopoulou M, Dimopoulos MA. Pathogenesis of bone disease in multiple myeloma: from bench to bedside. Blood Cancer J. 2018;8(1):7.
17. Schwarzer R, Nickel N, Godau J, Willie BM, Duda GN, Schwarzer R, et al. Notch pathway inhibition controls myeloma bone disease in the murine MOPC315.BM model. Blood Cancer J. 2014;4:e217.
18. Sanderson RD, Yang Y. Syndecan-1: a dynamic regulator of the myeloma microenvironment. Clin Exp Metastasis. 2008;25(2):149–59.
19. Novack DV, Mbalaviele G. Osteoclasts-key players in skeletal health and disease. Microbiol Spectr. 2016;4(3):1–19.
20. Bruns I, Cadeddu RP, Brueckmann I, Frobel J, Geyh S, Bust S, et al. Multiple myeloma-related deregulation of bone marrow-derived CD34(+) hematopoietic stem and progenitor cells. Blood. 2012;120(13):2620–30.
21. Bataille R, Chappard D, Basle MF. Quantifiable excess of bone resorption in monoclonal gammopathy is an early symptom of malignancy: a prospective study of 87 bone biopsies. Blood. 1996;87(11):4762–9.
22. Terpos E, Dimopoulos MA. Interaction between the skeletal and immune systems in cancer: mechanisms and clinical implications. Cancer Immunol Immunother. 2011;60(3):305–17.
23. Jakob C, Goerke A, Terpos E, Sterz J, Heider U, Kuhnhardt D, et al. Serum levels of total-RANKL in multiple myeloma. Clin Lymphoma Myeloma. 2009;9(6):430–5.
24. Politou M, Terpos E, Anagnostopoulos A, Szydlo R, Laffan M, Layton M, et al. Role of receptor activator of nuclear factor-kappa B ligand (RANKL), osteoprotegerin and macrophage protein 1-alpha (MIP-1a) in monoclonal gammopathy of undetermined significance (MGUS). Br J Haematol. 2004;126(5):686–9.
25. Goranova-Marinova V, Goranov S, Pavlov P, Tzvetkova T. Serum levels of OPG, RANKL and RANKL/OPG ratio in

newly-diagnosed patients with multiple myeloma. Clinical correlations. Haematologica. 2007;92(7):1000–1.
26. Terpos E, Christoulas D, Gavriatopoulou M, Dimopoulos MA. Mechanisms of bone destruction in multiple myeloma. Eur J Cancer Care (Engl). 2017;26(6):e12761.
27. Sezer O, Heider U, Jakob C, Eucker J, Possinger K. Human bone marrow myeloma cells express RANKL. J Clin Oncol. 2002;20(1):353–4.
28. Lai FP, Cole-Sinclair M, Cheng WJ, Quinn JM, Gillespie MT, Sentry JW, et al. Myeloma cells can directly contribute to the pool of RANKL in bone bypassing the classic stromal and osteoblast pathway of osteoclast stimulation. Br J Haematol. 2004;126(2):192–201.
29. Pearse RN, Sordillo EM, Yaccoby S, Wong BR, Liau DF, Colman N, et al. Multiple myeloma disrupts the TRANCE/osteoprotegerin cytokine axis to trigger bone destruction and promote tumor progression. Proc Natl Acad Sci U S A. 2001;98(20):11581–6.
30. Croucher PI, Shipman CM, Lippitt J, Perry M, Asosingh K, Hijzen A, et al. Osteoprotegerin inhibits the development of osteolytic bone disease in multiple myeloma. Blood. 2001;98(13):3534–40.
31. Henry DH, Costa L, Goldwasser F, Hirsh V, Hungria V, Prausova J, et al. Randomized, double-blind study of denosumab versus zoledronic acid in the treatment of bone metastases in patients with advanced cancer (excluding breast and prostate cancer) or multiple myeloma. J Clin Oncol. 2011;29(9):1125–32.
32. Standal T, Seidel C, Hjertner O, Plesner T, Sanderson RD, Waage A, et al. Osteoprotegerin is bound, internalized, and degraded by multiple myeloma cells. Blood. 2002;100(8):3002–7.
33. Abe M, Hiura K, Wilde J, Moriyama K, Hashimoto T, Ozaki S, et al. Role for macrophage inflammatory protein (MIP)-1alpha and MIP-1beta in the development of osteolytic lesions in multiple myeloma. Blood. 2002;100(6):2195–202.
34. Terpos E, Politou M, Szydlo R, Goldman JM, Apperley JF, Rahemtulla A. Serum levels of macrophage inflammatory protein-1 alpha (MIP-1alpha) correlate with the extent of bone disease and survival in patients with multiple myeloma. Br J Haematol. 2003;123(1):106–9.
35. Palma BD, Guasco D, Pedrazzoni M, Bolzoni M, Accardi F, Costa F, et al. Osteolytic lesions, cytogenetic features and bone marrow levels of cytokines and chemokines in multiple myeloma

patients: role of chemokine (C-C motif) ligand 20. Leukemia. 2016;30(2):409–16.
36. Choi SJ, Oba T, Callander NS, Jelinek DF, Roodman GD. AML-1A and AML-1B regulation of MIP-1alpha expression in multiple myeloma. Blood. 2003;101(10):3778–83.
37. Han JH, Choi SJ, Kurihara N, Koide M, Oba Y, Roodman GD. Macrophage inflammatory protein-1alpha is an osteoclastogenic factor in myeloma that is independent of receptor activator of nuclear factor kappaB ligand. Blood. 2001;97(11):3349–53.
38. Munshi N. Early evidence of anabolic bone activity of BHQ880, a fully human anti-DKK1 neutralizing antibody: results of a phase 2 study in previously untreated patients with smoldering multiple myeloma at risk for progression. Blood. 2012;120(21):331.
39. Noonan K, Marchionni L, Anderson J, Pardoll D, Roodman GD, Borrello I. A novel role of IL-17-producing lymphocytes in mediating lytic bone disease in multiple myeloma. Blood. 2010;116(18):3554–63.
40. Choi SJ, Cruz JC, Craig F, Chung H, Devlin RD, Roodman GD, et al. Macrophage inflammatory protein 1-alpha is a potential osteoclast stimulatory factor in multiple myeloma. Blood. 2000;96(2):671–5.
41. Dairaghi DJ, Oyajobi BO, Gupta A, McCluskey B, Miao S, Powers JP, et al. CCR1 blockade reduces tumor burden and osteolysis in vivo in a mouse model of myeloma bone disease. Blood. 2012;120(7):1449–57.
42. Giuliani N, Lisignoli G, Colla S, Lazzaretti M, Storti P, Mancini C, et al. CC-chemokine ligand 20/macrophage inflammatory protein-3alpha and CC-chemokine receptor 6 are overexpressed in myeloma microenvironment related to osteolytic bone lesions. Cancer Res. 2008;68(16):6840–50.
43. Kurihara N, Bertolini D, Suda T, Akiyama Y, Roodman GD. IL-6 stimulates osteoclast-like multinucleated cell formation in long term human marrow cultures by inducing IL-1 release. J Immunol. 1990;144(11):4226–30.
44. Kyrstsonis MC, Dedoussis G, Baxevanis C, Stamatelou M, Maniatis A. Serum interleukin-6 (IL-6) and interleukin-4 (IL-4) in patients with multiple myeloma (MM). Br J Haematol. 1996;92(2):420–2.
45. Kudo O, Sabokbar A, Pocock A, Itonaga I, Fujikawa Y, Athanasou NA. Interleukin-6 and interleukin-11 support human osteoclast formation by a RANKL-independent mechanism. Bone. 2003;32(1):1–7.

46. Fulciniti M, Hideshima T, Vermot-Desroches C, Pozzi S, Nanjappa P, Shen Z, et al. A high-affinity fully human anti-IL-6 mAb, 1339, for the treatment of multiple myeloma. Clin Cancer Res. 2009;15(23):7144–52.
47. Lee JW, Chung HY, Ehrlich LA, Jelinek DF, Callander NS, Roodman GD, et al. IL-3 expression by myeloma cells increases both osteoclast formation and growth of myeloma cells. Blood. 2004;103(6):2308–15.
48. Donovan KA, Lacy MQ, Gertz MA, Lust JA. IL-1beta expression in IgM monoclonal gammopathy and its relationship to multiple myeloma. Leukemia. 2002;16(3):382–5.
49. Lacy MQ, Donovan KA, Heimbach JK, Ahmann GJ, Lust JA. Comparison of interleukin-1 beta expression by in situ hybridization in monoclonal gammopathy of undetermined significance and multiple myeloma. Blood. 1999;93(1):300–5.
50. Yamamoto I, Kawano M, Sone T, Iwato K, Tanaka H, Ishikawa H, et al. Production of interleukin 1 beta, a potent bone resorbing cytokine, by cultured human myeloma cells. Cancer Res. 1989;49(15):4242–6.
51. Stromme O, Psonka-Antonczyk KM, Stokke BT, Sundan A, Arum CJ, Brede G. Myeloma-derived extracellular vesicles mediate HGF/c-Met signaling in osteoblast-like cells. Exp Cell Res. 2019;383(1):111490.
52. Kumar S, Witzig TE, Timm M, Haug J, Wellik L, Fonseca R, et al. Expression of VEGF and its receptors by myeloma cells. Leukemia. 2003;17(10):2025–31.
53. Tanaka Y, Abe M, Hiasa M, Oda A, Amou H, Nakano A, et al. Myeloma cell-osteoclast interaction enhances angiogenesis together with bone resorption: a role for vascular endothelial cell growth factor and osteopontin. Clin Cancer Res. 2007;13(3):816–23.
54. Bellamy WT. Expression of vascular endothelial growth factor and its receptors in multiple myeloma and other hematopoietic malignancies. Semin Oncol. 2001;28(6):551–9.
55. Standal T, Hjorth-Hansen H, Rasmussen T, Dahl IM, Lenhoff S, Brenne AT, et al. Osteopontin is an adhesive factor for myeloma cells and is found in increased levels in plasma from patients with multiple myeloma. Haematologica. 2004;89(2):174–82.
56. Valkovic T, Babarovic E, Lucin K, Stifter S, Aralica M, Pecanic S, et al. Plasma levels of osteopontin and vascular endothelial growth factor in association with clinical features and

parameters of tumor burden in patients with multiple myeloma. Biomed Res Int. 2014;2014:513170.
57. Cafforio P, Savonarola A, Stucci S, De Matteo M, Tucci M, Brunetti AE, et al. PTHrP produced by myeloma plasma cells regulates their survival and pro-osteoclast activity for bone disease progression. J Bone Miner Res. 2014;29(1):55–66.
58. Zannettino AC, Farrugia AN, Kortesidis A, Manavis J, To LB, Martin SK, et al. Elevated serum levels of stromal-derived factor-1alpha are associated with increased osteoclast activity and osteolytic bone disease in multiple myeloma patients. Cancer Res. 2005;65(5):1700–9.
59. Liu Y, Liang HM, Lv YQ, Tang SM, Cheng P. Blockade of SDF-1/CXCR4 reduces adhesion-mediated chemoresistance of multiple myeloma cells via interacting with interleukin-6. J Cell Physiol. 2019;234(11):19702–14.
60. Colucci S, Brunetti G, Mori G, Oranger A, Centonze M, Mori C, et al. Soluble decoy receptor 3 modulates the survival and formation of osteoclasts from multiple myeloma bone disease patients. Leukemia. 2009;23(11):2139–46.
61. Hemingway F, Taylor R, Knowles HJ, Athanasou NA. RANKL-independent human osteoclast formation with APRIL, BAFF, NGF, IGF I and IGF II. Bone. 2011;48(4):938–44.
62. Tai YT, Li XF, Breitkreutz I, Song W, Neri P, Catley L, et al. Role of B-cell-activating factor in adhesion and growth of human multiple myeloma cells in the bone marrow microenvironment. Cancer Res. 2006;66(13):6675–82.
63. Pan J, Sun Y, Zhang N, Li J, Ta F, Wei W, et al. Characteristics of BAFF and APRIL factor expression in multiple myeloma and clinical significance. Oncol Lett. 2017;14(3):2657–62.
64. Mohammad KS, Chen CG, Balooch G, Stebbins E, McKenna CR, Davis H, et al. Pharmacologic inhibition of the TGF-beta type I receptor kinase has anabolic and anti-catabolic effects on bone. PLoS One. 2009;4(4):e5275.
65. Terpos E, Kastritis E, Christoulas D, Gkotzamanidou M, Eleutherakis-Papaiakovou E, Kanellias N, et al. Circulating activin-A is elevated in patients with advanced multiple myeloma and correlates with extensive bone involvement and inferior survival; no alterations post-lenalidomide and dexamethasone therapy. Ann Oncol. 2012;23(10):2681–6.
66. Sugatani T, Alvarez UM, Hruska KA. Activin A stimulates IkappaB-alpha/NFkappaB and RANK expression for osteoclast

differentiation, but not AKT survival pathway in osteoclast precursors. J Cell Biochem. 2003;90(1):59–67.
67. Fuller K, Bayley KE, Chambers TJ. Activin A is an essential cofactor for osteoclast induction. Biochem Biophys Res Commun. 2000;268(1):2–7.
68. Pitari MR, Rossi M, Amodio N, Botta C, Morelli E, Federico C, et al. Inhibition of miR-21 restores RANKL/OPG ratio in multiple myeloma-derived bone marrow stromal cells and impairs the resorbing activity of mature osteoclasts. Oncotarget. 2015;6(29):27343–58.
69. Brunetti G, Oranger A, Mori G, Centonze M, Colaianni G, Rizzi R, et al. The formation of osteoclasts in multiple myeloma bone disease patients involves the secretion of soluble decoy receptor 3. Ann N Y Acad Sci. 2010;1192:298–302.
70. Gavriatopoulou M, Dimopoulos MA, Christoulas D, Migkou M, Iakovaki M, Gkotzamanidou M, et al. Dickkopf-1: a suitable target for the management of myeloma bone disease. Expert Opin Ther Targets. 2009;13(7):839–48.
71. McDonald MM, Reagan MR, Youlten SE, Mohanty ST, Seckinger A, Terry RL, et al. Inhibiting the osteocyte-specific protein sclerostin increases bone mass and fracture resistance in multiple myeloma. Blood. 2017;129(26):3452–64.
72. Tjin EP, Derksen PW, Kataoka H, Spaargaren M, Pals ST. Multiple myeloma cells catalyze hepatocyte growth factor (HGF) activation by secreting the serine protease HGF-activator. Blood. 2004;104(7):2172–5.
73. Hjertner O, Torgersen ML, Seidel C, Hjorth-Hansen H, Waage A, Borset M, et al. Hepatocyte growth factor (HGF) induces interleukin-11 secretion from osteoblasts: a possible role for HGF in myeloma-associated osteolytic bone disease. Blood. 1999;94(11):3883–8.
74. Seidel C, Borset M, Turesson I, Abildgaard N, Sundan A, Waage A. Elevated serum concentrations of hepatocyte growth factor in patients with multiple myeloma. The Nordic Myeloma Study Group. Blood. 1998;91(3):806–12.
75. Pfeilschifter J, Chenu C, Bird A, Mundy GR, Roodman GD. Interleukin-1 and tumor necrosis factor stimulate the formation of human osteoclastlike cells in vitro. J Bone Miner Res. 1989;4(1):113–8.
76. Roodman GD. Pathogenesis of myeloma bone disease. Leukemia. 2009;23(3):435–41.

77. Silbermann R, Bolzoni M, Storti P, Guasco D, Bonomini S, Zhou D, et al. Bone marrow monocyte–/macrophage-derived activin A mediates the osteoclastogenic effect of IL-3 in multiple myeloma. Leukemia. 2014;28(4):951–4.
78. Xi H, An R, Li L, Wang G, Tao Y, Gao L. Myeloma bone disease: progress in pathogenesis. Prog Biophys Mol Biol. 2016;122(2):149–55.
79. Robbiani DF, Colon K, Ely S, Ely S, Chesi M, Bergsagel PL. Osteopontin dysregulation and lytic bone lesions in multiple myeloma. Hematol Oncol. 2007;25(1):16–20.
80. Roux S, Mariette X. The high rate of bone resorption in multiple myeloma is due to RANK (receptor activator of nuclear factor-kappaB) and RANK ligand expression. Leuk Lymphoma. 2004;45(6):1111–8.
81. Bouyssou JM, Ghobrial IM, Roccaro AM. Targeting SDF-1 in multiple myeloma tumor microenvironment. Cancer Lett. 2016;380(1):315–8.
82. Beider K, Begin M, Abraham M, Wald H, Weiss ID, Wald O, et al. CXCR4 antagonist 4F-benzoyl-TN14003 inhibits leukemia and multiple myeloma tumor growth. Exp Hematol. 2011;39(3):282–92.
83. Lam J, Takeshita S, Barker JE, Kanagawa O, Ross FP, Teitelbaum SL. TNF-alpha induces osteoclastogenesis by direct stimulation of macrophages exposed to permissive levels of RANK ligand. J Clin Invest. 2000;106(12):1481–8.
84. Hongming H, Jian H. Bortezomib inhibits maturation and function of osteoclasts from PBMCs of patients with multiple myeloma by downregulating TRAF6. Leuk Res. 2009;33(1):115–22.
85. Chen H, Li M, Sanchez E, Wang CS, Lee T, Soof CM, et al. Combined TRAF6 targeting and proteasome blockade has anti-myeloma and anti-bone resorptive effects. Mol Cancer Res. 2017;15(5):598–609.
86. Liu H, Tamashiro S, Baritaki S, Penichet M, Yu Y, Chen H, et al. TRAF6 activation in multiple myeloma: a potential therapeutic target. Clin Lymphoma Myeloma Leuk. 2012;12(3):155–63.
87. Xu G, Liu K, Anderson J, Patrene K, Lentzsch S, Roodman GD, et al. Expression of XBP1s in bone marrow stromal cells is critical for myeloma cell growth and osteoclast formation. Blood. 2012;119(18):4205–14.

Chapter 3
The Pathophysiology of Myeloma Bone Disease: Role of Osteoblasts and Osteocytes

Nicola Giuliani, Federica Costa, and Valentina Marchica

Introduction

Bone disease is the hallmark of multiple myeloma (MM) [1]. Plasma cell (PC) accumulation into the bone microenvironment leads to bone destruction due to a severe unbalanced and uncoupled bone remodeling [2, 3]. Indeed, an increased osteoclast (OCL) recruitment and activity together with a severe osteoblast (OB) suppression have been demonstrated in MM patients [2, 3].

N. Giuliani (✉)
Department of Medicine and Surgery, University of Parma, Parma, Italy

Hematology, "Azienda Ospedaliero-Universitaria di Parma", Parma, Italy
e-mail: nicola.giuliani@unipr.it

F. Costa · V. Marchica
Department of Medicine and Surgery, University of Parma, Parma, Italy

E. Zamagni (ed.), *Management of Bone Disease and Kidney Failure in Multiple Myeloma*,
https://doi.org/10.1007/978-3-030-63662-3_3

On the other hand, patients with premalignant monoclonal gammopathy, as monoclonal gammopathy of undetermined significance (MGUS) and smoldering MM, are characterized by an unbalanced but coupled bone remodeling with an increased OCL formation and activity that causes a higher risk of fractures without development of osteolytic lesions.

Osteolytic MM bone disease occurs in about 80% of MM patients at diagnosis [4], resulting in pathological fractures, spinal cord compression, and pain, significantly impacting their quality of life [2, 3].

Concerning the pathophysiology of MM bone disease, the cell-to-cell contact between MM and microenvironment cells is critically involved in the upregulation of several cytokines and chemokines, resulting in the stimulation of OCL formation and activity along with the inhibition of OB differentiation. These alterations of bone marrow (BM) microenvironment, which consequently lead to MM bone disease onset, provide a permissive niche that promotes growth and survival of MM cells [2, 3].

Pathophysiology of Myeloma-Induced Osteoblast Suppression

The relationship between MM cells and OBs is complex [5–7]. MM cells can induce suppression of osteoblastogenesis; in turn, OBs can affect MM cell growth [5–8].

The capacity of MM cells to suppress osteoblastic cells and their function is well known; this effect is the result of both impairment of OB formation, by blocking the osteogenic differentiation of MSCs and the inhibition of existing OBs [9–22].

The interaction between MM cells and MSCs inhibits the activity of Runt-related transcription factor 2 (Runx2), the main pro-osteoblastogenic transcription factor, in MSCs thus leading to the suppression of OB differentiation [23]. This effect may be due to the capacity of MM cells to upregulate growth factor independent protein (GFI)-1, a negative regulator of Runx2 activity that is overexpressed by BM-MSCs in MM patients. These effects are mediated, at least in part, by the cell-to-cell contact between MM and OB precursor (Pre-OB) cells. This cell-to-cell contact involves interactions between very late antigen-4 (VLA-4) on MM cells and vascular cell adhesion molecule 1 (VCAM-1) on OB progenitors, as demonstrated by the capacity of a neutralizing VLA-4 antibody to reduce the inhibitory effects of MM cells on Runx2/Cbfa1 activity [9]. The role of cell-to-cell contact via the VLA-4/VCAM-1 interaction in the development of bone lesions by OCL activation and OB inhibition in MM has been recently demonstrated using *in vivo* mouse models [24]. The implantation of the human MM cell line JJN3, with relatively high VLA-4 expression, in irradiated severe combined immunodeficient (SCID) mice, leads to the development of lytic lesions and marked osteoblastopenia, with a significant reduction of bone formation [25]. In addition to VLA-4/VCAM-1, other adhesion molecules appear to be involved in the inhibition of osteoblastogenesis by human MM cells. For example, neural cell adhesion molecule (NCAM) interaction between MM cells and MSC/osteoblastic cells decreases bone matrix production by osteoblastic cells and may contribute to the development of bone lesions in MM patients [26].

Soluble factors can be involved in the suppression of the osteogenic differentiation of stromal cells and the inhibition of Runx2 activity. MM patients show high BM levels of cytokines such as interleukin (IL)-7 and hepatocyte growth factor (HGF) that contribute to the Runx2 inhibition and osteoblastogenesis decrease [27, 28]. IL-7 reduces Runx2/Cbfa1 promoter activity and the expression of osteoblastic markers in OBs [29]. Moreover, IL-7 can inhibit bone formation *in vivo* in mice [30] as well as colony-forming unit (CFU)-fibroblast (F) and CFU-OB formation in human BM cultures, and it decreases Runx2 activity in human Pre-OBs [9]. The potential involvement of IL-7 in MM has been further supported by the finding of higher IL-7 plasma levels in MM patients compared to normal subjects, [31] and by the capacity of IL-7 blocking antibodies (Abs) to partially blunt the inhibitory effects of MM cells on OB differentiation [9].

HGF is produced by MM cells, and its high levels in the BM of MM patients correlated with those of alkaline phosphatase (ALP) [31]. HGF inhibits *in vitro* osteoblastogenesis induced by bone morphogenetic proteins (BMP)-2 and BMP-induced expression of ALP in both human and murine stromal cells. Moreover, the expression of the transcription factors Runx2 and osterix (Osx), in addition to small mother against decapentaplegic (Smad), is reduced by HGF treatment [31]. Transforming growth factors (TGF)-β, a multifunctional protein released from the bone matrix during osteoclastic bone resorption, inhibits OB differentiation. In addition to reduced myeloma growth, inhibition of TGF-β signaling has been shown to block the ability of myeloma cells to inhibit OB differentiation *in vitro* [32]. TAZ, a Runx2/Cbfa1 transcriptional coactivator, has recently been shown to modulate the osteogenic potential of human MSCs (hMSCs) and to be expressed at lower levels in MM patients compared to healty donors (HDs) [33]. The repressed osteogenesis and TAZ expression were both partially restored by neutralization of tumor necrosis factor (TNF)-α [34].

The potential involvement of inhibitors of Wnt signaling in the suppression of OB formation and function in MM has been also investigated. Primary CD138$^+$ MM cells overexpress the Wnt inhibitor dickkopf-related protein-1 *(DKK1)* compared to normal PCs and those from patients with MGUS [35]. Gene expression profiling has demonstrated a tight correlation between *DKK1* expression by MM cells and the occurrence of focal lytic bone lesions in MM patients; moreover, high DKK1 levels in BM and peripheral sera in MM patients correlate with the presence of bone lesions [36]. Another work has shown that MM cells produce other Wnt inhibitors, including secreted frizzled-related protein (SFRP)3/frizzled-related protein *(FRZB)*. *FRZB* is highly expressed by CD138$^+$ MM cells compared to PCs from MGUS patients, and BM plasma levels are higher in MM patients with bone lesions compared to MM patients without skeletal involvement [36]. SFRP2 has been also reported to be produced by some human MM cell lines and by patients with advanced MM bone disease; [37] SFRP2 can inhibit OB differentiation of murine Pre-OBs [37]. Canonical Wnt signaling, however, is not suppressed in MM-derived hMSCs and Pre-OBs [9, 36].

In vivo evidences suggest that DKK1 and canonical Wnt signaling are potential targets in MM bone microenvironment. Canonical Wnt signaling activation leads to bone mass improvement by reducing the development of osteolytic lesions in MM mouse models [37–40]. Activated Wnt signaling in OBs by treatment with lithium chloride inhibited MM bone disease and decreased tumor burden in the bone [38]. Other *in vivo* mouse models, such as SCID-humanized (hu) mice, used to evaluate the role of osteoblastic cells in the development of osteolytic lesions, showed that the stimulation of osteoblastic cells reduces *in vitro* MM cell growth in the presence of OCLs [18] and that blocking DKK1 increases bone formation and bone mass [41].

It has been recently shown that the activation of the non-canonical signal pathway by Wnt5a, mediated by the Receptor Tyrosine Kinase Like Orphan Receptor (ROR)2 receptor rather than activation of the canonical pathway by Wnt3a, stimulates differentiation of osteoblast CFU-OB precursors in human BM cultures [42–44].

Recently, our experimental data suggested that MM cells inhibit non-canonical Wnt signaling in Pre-OB cells, including the Wnt5a/Ca^{2+}/PKC and Wnt5a/ROR2 transduction pathways, thus inhibiting the activity of both Nuclear Factor Of Activated T Cells (NFATc)1 and Rho-associated protein kinase (ROCK). The capacity of MM cells to inhibit *ROR2* expression and non-canonical Wnt signaling in human PreOB cells was observed both in the presence and absence of a transwell insert [45], as we have previously reported for Runx2 activity [9]. This suggests that both soluble factors and cell-to-cell contact may be involved. Interestingly, it has been reported that the Runx2 and Wnt5a/ROR2 pathways have a cooperative rather than direct relationship in controlling osteoblastogenesis [46, 47], which supports the hypothesis that both systems are probably involved in the MM-induced suppression of osteogenic differentiation of BM-MSCs. In addition, the activation of non-canonical Wnt signaling in hMSCs by Wnt5a and the overexpression of either Wnt5 or ROR2 by lentivirus vectors increased the osteogenic differentiation of hMSCs and blunted the inhibitory effect of MM cells in co-culture. Wnt5a inhibition by specific small interfering RNA (siRNA) also reduced the BM hMSC expression of osteogenic markers [45]. These findings demonstrate that the Wnt5a/ROR2 pathway is involved in the pathophysiology of MM-induced OB suppression and that the activation of the non-canonical Wnt5a/ROR2 pathway in BM hMSCs increases the osteogenic differentiation and may counterbalance the inhibitory effect of MM cells.

Impaired OB formation in MM is also associated with a blockade of deactivation of Notch signaling. Active in MM cells, the Notch pathway results in increased proliferation, resistance to apoptosis, and pro-osteoclastogenic activity [48]. Recently, it has been reported that blocking Notch signaling significantly reduces BM homing and infiltration of MM cells through the involvement of the C-X-C chemokine receptor type (CXCR)4–C-X-C Motif Chemokine Ligand (CXCL)12 axis in the BM [49]. Notch activation in MM cells occurs either through the co-expression of the Notch 1–3 receptors and their ligands Jagged 1–2 resulting in an autocrine pathway activation, or through the trigger of MSCs that express Delta-like or Jagged ligands [48]. Interestingly, it has been reported that Notch signaling is downregulated during osteogenesis in hMSCs, whereas in MM patients, Notch signaling is highly activated in relation to the suppression of hMSC osteoblastic differentiation [50]. The blockade of Notch signaling by either a γ-secretase drug inhibitor or a Notch-specific siRNA enhances Runx2 expression and the osteogenic properties in hMSCs, restoring the osteogenic differentiation properties of MSCs in MM patients [50].

Role of Exosomes in the Pathophysiology of MM-Induced OB Suppression

Extracellular vesicles (EVs), which include exosomes and microvesicles (MVs), are endosomal-derived vesicles secreted by several types of cells for transporting proteins, lipids, and nucleic acids, such as microRNAs (miRs) and messenger RNAs (mRNAs), between cells.

Emerging evidence indicates that EVs function as intercellular communicators among the bone cells within BM microenvironment, both in physiological processes and pathological conditions. A number of reports highlighted the crucial role of miRs in controlling OCL and OB activity [51].

Recent studies have shown that miRs are involved in osteogenic lineage commitment by targeting the components of bone formation pathways [23, 27, 28, 52, 53]. In a recent work, using a miR array approach, the authors showed that miR-135b was upregulated in MM MSCs compared to HD MSCs and that the miR-135b relative expression was inversely correlated to ALP activity, suggesting a possible role in the osteogenic differentiation impairment [28]. The effects of miR-135b on osteogenic differentiation were confirmed by using both a miR-135b inhibitor and a mimetic and then demonstrating the modulation of osteogenic markers. Finally, in a co-culture system between MM cells and HD MSCs it was reported that a soluble factor produced by MM cells stimulated the upregulation of miR-135b by HD MSCs [28].

Osteocytes and Myeloma Bone Disease

Recently, the interplay between MM cells and osteocytes and their role in MM bone disease have been underlined. Eisenberger et al. [54] presented a transcriptome analysis of the *in vivo* effects of MM cells on osteocytes. The study clearly demonstrated that MM-induced stress generated specific gene expression footprints in osteocytes [54]. More recently, a histological study performed on human bone biopsies revealed that MM patients were characterized by increased osteocyte death and fewer viable osteocytes when compared with healthy controls [55]. Moreover, the presence of osteolysis in MM patients correlated with the increased osteocyte death, probably due to an increased osteocyte apoptosis. Interestingly, MM patients, when compared to healthy controls or MGUS patients, showed a higher number of OCLs negatively correlating with the number of viable osteocytes. The same study showed that in a co-culture system, MM cells upregulated the production of pro-osteoclastogenic molecules such as IL-11, matrix metalloproteinase (MMP)-1, and chemokine (C-C motif) ligand (CCL)3/macrophage inflammatory protein (MIP)-1α by preosteocytes [55]. Indeed, the conditioned media of these co-cultures increased the *in vitro* OCL formation that was inhibited by the presence of anti-CCL3 and anti-IL-11 antibodies. The immunohistochemical analysis of bone biopsies showed that the osteocytic expression of IL-11 was higher in osteolytic MM patients when compared to non-osteolytic ones, even though there were no differences between MM and MGUS patients. Later, the same group demonstrated that MM cells induced autophagic cell death in co-cultured osteocytes, thus supporting the notion that other mechanisms, other than apoptosis, underlie the role of osteocytes in MM bone disease [56].

Osteocytes are in direct contact with MM cells in MM-bearing mice, and so, these interactions increase apoptosis and the production of receptor activator of nuclear factor kappa-β ligand (RANKL) and sclerostin (Scl) by osteocytes [57]. *In vitro* experiments demonstrated that the activation of Notch signaling underlined the increased osteocytic apoptosis resulting in [1] increased expression of RANKL and ability of osteocytes to recruit OCL precursors and [2] increased production of Scl, which in turn inhibits Wnt signaling and OB differentiation. Of note, this physical interaction induces the reciprocal activation of Notch pathway in osteocytes and MM cells, supporting the growth and proliferation of tumor cells [57]. One of the possible MM factors responsible for the increased osteocyte death was TNF-α, as recombinant TNF-α increased osteocyte apoptosis and neutralizing anti-human TNF-α antibody blocked the MM-induced reduction of osteocyte viability [57]. Together these data suggest that, in MM-colonized bone, osteocytes are responsible for the increased OCL recruitment as well as the inhibition of bone formation through cell-to-cell interactions and release of soluble factors.

Conclusion

The pathophysiology of MM-induced bone disease is complex and involves several mechanisms. OB inhibition and OCL activation are mainly triggered by the high RANKL/osteoprotegerin (OPG) ratio in BM microenvironment, through the cell-to-cell contact.

OB formation is impaired by the block of osteogenic differentiation of BM MSCs, through the inhibition of the Runx2 activity mediated by different mechanisms. The deregulation of Wnt-signaling in MM cells and in BM MSCs is also involved in the suppression of OB formation.

More recently, studies underline the role of exosomes and MVs that transport several miRs and mRNAs in the regulation of OCL formation and the osteogenic differentiation of MSCs. Actually, their pathophysiological role in MM-induced bone disease is under investigation. Interestingly, it has been shown that miR-135b is upregulated in MM MSCs compared to HD MSCs and that the miR-135b relative expression was inversely correlated to ALP activity, suggesting a possible role in the osteogenic differentiation impairment.

Finally, the role of osteocytes in the development of bone remodeling alterations in MM has been demonstrated showing that MM cells induce osteocyte death by apoptosis and autophagy triggering in turn the production of pro-osteoclastogenic cytokines and inhibitors of bone formation as scl.

Figure 3.1 summarizes the main pathophysiological mechanisms involved in MM-induced bone destruction focusing on the role of OBs and osteocytes.

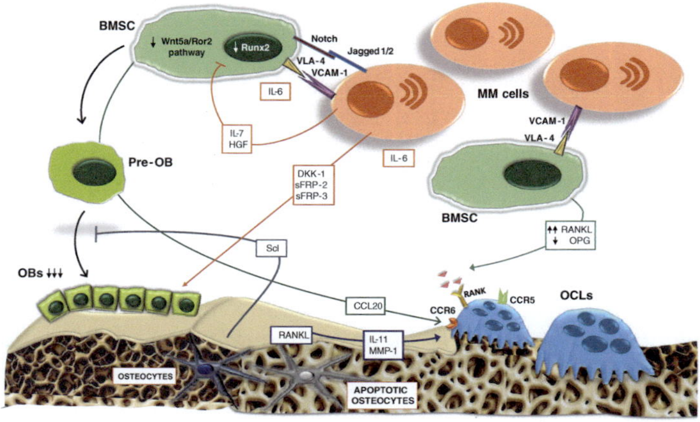

FIGURE 3.1 Pathophysiology of myeloma-induced bone disease. Mechanisms involved in MM-induced OB inhibition. Role of the cell-to-cell contact between MM cells and BM MSC in the block of the osteogenic differentiation of MSCs. Osteocytes are also involved in MM-induced OB inhibition by scl and osteoclast OCL formation. Abbreviations: BMSC bone marrow mesenchymal stromal cells, CCL chemokine (C-C motif) ligand, CCR C-C chemokine receptor, DKK dickkopf-related protein, HGF hepatocyte growth factor, IL interleukin, IFN interferon, MMP metalloproteinase, MM multiple myeloma, OB osteoblast, Pre-OB OB precursor, OCL osteoclast, OPG osteoprotegerin, RANKL receptor-activated nuclear factor–κB ligand, ROR Receptor tyrosine kinase-like orphan, Runx runt-related transcription factor, Scl sclerostin, sFRP secreted frizzled-related protein, TNF tumor necrosis factor, VCAM vascular cell adhesion molecule, VLA very late antigen

References

1. Palumbo A, Anderson K. Multiple myeloma. N Engl J Med. 2011;364(11):1046–60.
2. Roodman GD. Pathogenesis of myeloma bone disease. Leukemia. 2009;23(3):435–41.
3. Yaccoby S. Advances in the understanding of myeloma bone disease and tumour growth. Br J Haematol. 2010;149(3):311–21.

4. Kyle RA, Gertz MA, Witzig TE, Lust JA, Lacy MQ, Dispenzieri A, et al. Review of 1027 patients with newly diagnosed multiple myeloma. Mayo Clin Proc. 2003;78(1):21–33.
5. Giuliani N, Mangoni M, Rizzoli V. Osteogenic differentiation of mesenchymal stem cells in multiple myeloma: identification of potential therapeutic targets. Exp Hematol. 2009;37(8):879–86.
6. Giuliani N, Rizzoli V, Roodman GD. Multiple myeloma bone disease: pathophysiology of osteoblast inhibition. Blood. 2006;108(13):3992–6.
7. Roodman GD. Osteoblast function in myeloma. Bone. 2011;48(1):135–40.
8. Yaccoby S. Osteoblastogenesis and tumor growth in myeloma. Leuk Lymphoma. 2010;51(2):213–20.
9. Giuliani N, Colla S, Morandi F, Lazzaretti M, Sala R, Bonomini S, et al. Myeloma cells block RUNX2/CBFA1 activity in human bone marrow osteoblast progenitors and inhibit osteoblast formation and differentiation. Blood. 2005;106(7):2472–83.
10. Garayoa M, Garcia JL, Santamaria C, Garcia-Gomez A, Blanco JF, Pandiella A, et al. Mesenchymal stem cells from multiple myeloma patients display distinct genomic profile as compared with those from normal donors. Leukemia. 2009;23(8):1515–27.
11. Gainor BJ, Buchert P. Fracture healing in metastatic bone disease. Clin Orthop Relat Res. 1983;178:297–302.
12. Giuliani N, Lisignoli G, Novara F, Storti P, Zaffaroni N, Villa R, et al. Bone osteoblastic and mesenchymal stromal cells lack primarily tumoral features in multiple myeloma patients. Leukemia. 2010;24(7):1368–70.
13. Reagan MR, Mishima Y, Glavey SV, Zhang Y, Manier S, Lu ZN, et al. Investigating osteogenic differentiation in multiple myeloma using a novel 3D bone marrow niche model. Blood. 2014;124(22):3250–9.
14. Lokhorst HM, Lamme T, de Smet M, Klein S, de Weger RA, van Oers R, et al. Primary tumor cells of myeloma patients induce interleukin-6 secretion in long-term bone marrow cultures. Blood. 1994;84(7):2269–77.
15. Li B, Fu J, Chen P, Zhuang W. Impairment in immunomodulatory function of mesenchymal stem cells from multiple myeloma patients. Arch Med Res. 2010;41(8):623–33.
16. Corre J, Mahtouk K, Attal M, Gadelorge M, Huynh A, Fleury-Cappellesso S, et al. Bone marrow mesenchymal stem cells are abnormal in multiple myeloma. Leukemia. 2007;21(5):1079–88.

17. Wang J, Hendrix A, Hernot S, Lemaire M, De Bruyne E, Van Valckenborgh E, et al. Bone marrow stromal cell-derived exosomes as communicators in drug resistance in multiple myeloma cells. Blood. 2014;124(4):555–66.
18. Yaccoby S, Wezeman MJ, Zangari M, Walker R, Cottler-Fox M, Gaddy D, et al. Inhibitory effects of osteoblasts and increased bone formation on myeloma in novel culture systems and a myelomatous mouse model. Haematologica. 2006;91(2):192–9.
19. Wallace SR, Oken MM, Lunetta KL, Panoskaltsis-Mortari A, Masellis AM. Abnormalities of bone marrow mesenchymal cells in multiple myeloma patients. Cancer. 2001;91(7):1219–30.
20. Arnulf B, Lecourt S, Soulier J, Ternaux B, Lacassagne MN, Crinquette A, et al. Phenotypic and functional characterization of bone marrow mesenchymal stem cells derived from patients with multiple myeloma. Leukemia. 2007;21(1):158–63.
21. Silvestris F, Lombardi L, De Matteo M, Bruno A, Dammacco F. Myeloma bone disease: pathogenetic mechanisms and clinical assessment. Leuk Res. 2007;31(2):129–38.
22. Kassen D, Moore S, Percy L, Herledan G, Bounds D, Rodriguez-Justo M, et al. The bone marrow stromal compartment in multiple myeloma patients retains capability for osteogenic differentiation in vitro: defining the stromal defect in myeloma. Br J Haematol. 2014;167(2):194–206.
23. Kim KM, Park SJ, Jung SH, Kim EJ, Jogeswar G, Ajita J, et al. miR-182 is a negative regulator of osteoblast proliferation, differentiation, and skeletogenesis through targeting FoxO1. J Bone Miner Res. 2012;27(8):1669–79.
24. Mori Y, Shimizu N, Dallas M, Niewolna M, Story B, Williams PJ, et al. Anti-alpha4 integrin antibody suppresses the development of multiple myeloma and associated osteoclastic osteolysis. Blood. 2004;104(7):2149–54.
25. Hjorth-Hansen H, Seifert MF, Borset M, Aarset H, Ostlie A, Sundan A, et al. Marked osteoblastopenia and reduced bone formation in a model of multiple myeloma bone disease in severe combined immunodeficiency mice. J Bone Miner Res Off J Am Soc Bone Miner Res. 1999;14(2):256–63.
26. Ely SA, Knowles DM. Expression of CD56/neural cell adhesion molecule correlates with the presence of lytic bone lesions in multiple myeloma and distinguishes myeloma from monoclonal gammopathy of undetermined significance and lymphomas with plasmacytoid differentiation. Am J Pathol. 2002;160(4):1293–9.

27. Huang S, Wang S, Bian C, Yang Z, Zhou H, Zeng Y, et al. Upregulation of miR-22 promotes osteogenic differentiation and inhibits adipogenic differentiation of human adipose tissue-derived mesenchymal stem cells by repressing HDAC6 protein expression. Stem Cells Dev. 2012;21(13):2531–40.
28. Xu S, Cecilia Santini G, De Veirman K, Vande Broek I, Leleu X, De Becker A, et al. Upregulation of miR-135b is involved in the impaired osteogenic differentiation of mesenchymal stem cells derived from multiple myeloma patients. PLoS One. 2013;8(11):e79752.
29. Weitzmann MN, Roggia C, Toraldo G, Weitzmann L, Pacifici R. Increased production of IL-7 uncouples bone formation from bone resorption during estrogen deficiency. J Clin Invest. 2002;110(11):1643–50.
30. Giuliani N, Colla S, Sala R, Moroni M, Lazzaretti M, La Monica S, et al. Human myeloma cells stimulate the receptor activator of nuclear factor-kappa B ligand (RANKL) in T lymphocytes: a potential role in multiple myeloma bone disease. Blood. 2002;100(13):4615–21.
31. Standal T, Abildgaard N, Fagerli UM, Stordal B, Hjertner O, Borset M, et al. HGF inhibits BMP-induced osteoblastogenesis: possible implications for the bone disease of multiple myeloma. Blood. 2007;109(7):3024–30.
32. Edwards CM, Zhuang J, Mundy GR. The pathogenesis of the bone disease of multiple myeloma. Bone. 2008;42(6):1007–13.
33. Hong JH, Hwang ES, McManus MT, Amsterdam A, Tian Y, Kalmukova R, et al. TAZ, a transcriptional modulator of mesenchymal stem cell differentiation. Science. 2005;309(5737):1074–8.
34. Li B, Shi M, Li J, Zhang H, Chen B, Chen L, et al. Elevated tumor necrosis factor-alpha suppresses TAZ expression and impairs osteogenic potential of Flk-1+ mesenchymal stem cells in patients with multiple myeloma. Stem Cells Dev. 2007;16(6):921–30.
35. Tian E, Zhan F, Walker R, Rasmussen E, Ma Y, Barlogie B, et al. The role of the Wnt-signaling antagonist DKK1 in the development of osteolytic lesions in multiple myeloma. N Engl J Med. 2003;349(26):2483–94.
36. Giuliani N, Morandi F, Tagliaferri S, Lazzaretti M, Donofrio G, Bonomini S, et al. Production of Wnt inhibitors by myeloma cells: potential effects on canonical Wnt pathway in the bone microenvironment. Cancer Res. 2007;67(16):7665–74.

37. Oshima T, Abe M, Asano J, Hara T, Kitazoe K, Sekimoto E, et al. Myeloma cells suppress bone formation by secreting a soluble Wnt inhibitor, sFRP-2. Blood. 2005;106(9):3160–5.
38. Edwards CM, Edwards JR, Lwin ST, Esparza J, Oyajobi BO, McCluskey B, et al. Increasing Wnt signaling in the bone marrow microenvironment inhibits the development of myeloma bone disease and reduces tumor burden in bone in vivo. Blood. 2008;111(5):2833–42.
39. Qiang YW, Shaughnessy JD Jr, Yaccoby S. Wnt3a signaling within bone inhibits multiple myeloma bone disease and tumor growth. Blood. 2008;112(2):374–82.
40. Fulciniti M, Tassone P, Hideshima T, Vallet S, Nanjappa P, Ettenberg SA, et al. Anti-DKK1 mAb (BHQ880) as a potential therapeutic agent for multiple myeloma. Blood. 2009;114(2):371–9.
41. Yaccoby S, Ling W, Zhan F, Walker R, Barlogie B, Shaughnessy JD Jr. Antibody-based inhibition of DKK1 suppresses tumor-induced bone resorption and multiple myeloma growth in vivo. Blood. 2007;109(5):2106–11.
42. Liu Y, Rubin B, Bodine PV, Billiard J. Wnt5a induces homodimerization and activation of Ror2 receptor tyrosine kinase. J Cell Biochem. 2008;105(2):497–502.
43. Baksh D, Tuan RS. Canonical and non-canonical Wnts differentially affect the development potential of primary isolate of human bone marrow mesenchymal stem cells. J Cell Physiol. 2007;212(3):817–26.
44. Baksh D, Boland GM, Tuan RS. Cross-talk between Wnt signaling pathways in human mesenchymal stem cells leads to functional antagonism during osteogenic differentiation. J Cell Biochem. 2007;101(5):1109–24.
45. Bolzoni M, Donofrio G, Storti P, Guasco D, Toscani D, Lazzaretti M, et al. Myeloma cells inhibit non-canonical Wnt co-receptor ror2 expression in human bone marrow osteoprogenitor cells: effect of wnt5a/ror2 pathway activation on the osteogenic differentiation impairment induced by myeloma cells. Leukemia. 2013;27(2):451–63.
46. Koga T, Matsui Y, Asagiri M, Kodama T, de Crombrugghe B, Nakashima K, et al. NFAT and Osterix cooperatively regulate bone formation. Nat Med. 2005;11(8):880–5.
47. Penolazzi L, Lisignoli G, Lambertini E, Torreggiani E, Manferdini C, Lolli A, et al. Transcription factor decoy against NFATc1 in human primary osteoblasts. Int J Mol Med. 2011;28(2):199–206.

48. Colombo M, Mirandola L, Platonova N, Apicella L, Basile A, Figueroa AJ, et al. Notch-directed microenvironment reprogramming in myeloma: a single path to multiple outcomes. Leukemia. 2013;27(5):1009–18.
49. Mirandola L, Apicella L, Colombo M, Yu Y, Berta DG, Platonova N, et al. Anti-notch treatment prevents multiple myeloma cells localization to the bone marrow via the chemokine system CXCR4/SDF-1. Leukemia. 2013;27(7):1558–66.
50. Xu S, Evans H, Buckle C, De Veirman K, Hu J, Xu D, et al. Impaired osteogenic differentiation of mesenchymal stem cells derived from multiple myeloma patients is associated with a blockade in the deactivation of the notch signaling pathway. Leukemia. 2012;26(12):2546–9.
51. Shapiro IM, Landis WJ, Risbud MV. Matrix vesicles: are they anchored exosomes? Bone. 2015;79:29–36.
52. Wu T, Xie M, Wang X, Jiang X, Li J, Huang H. miR-155 modulates TNF-alpha-inhibited osteogenic differentiation by targeting SOCS1 expression. Bone. 2012;51(3):498–505.
53. Hu W, Ye Y, Zhang W, Wang J, Chen A, Guo F. miR1423p promotes osteoblast differentiation by modulating Wnt signaling. Mol Med Rep. 2013;7(2):689–93.
54. Eisenberger S, Ackermann K, Voggenreiter G, Sultmann H, Kasperk C, Pyerin W. Metastases and multiple myeloma generate distinct transcriptional footprints in osteocytes in vivo. J Pathol. 2008;214(5):617–26.
55. Giuliani N, Ferretti M, Bolzoni M, Storti P, Lazzaretti M, Dalla Palma B, et al. Increased osteocyte death in multiple myeloma patients: role in myeloma-induced osteoclast formation. Leukemia. 2012;26(6):1391–401.
56. Toscani D, Palumbo C, Dalla Palma B, Ferretti M, Bolzoni M, Marchica V, et al. The proteasome inhibitor Bortezomib maintains osteocyte viability in multiple myeloma patients by reducing both apoptosis and autophagy: a new function for proteasome inhibitors. J Bone Miner Res Off J Am Soc Bone Miner Res. 2016;31(4):815–27.
57. Delgado-Calle J, Anderson J, Cregor MD, Hiasa M, Chirgwin JM, Carlesso N, et al. Bidirectional notch signaling and osteocyte-derived factors in the bone marrow microenvironment promote tumor cell proliferation and bone destruction in multiple myeloma. Cancer Res. 2016;76(5):1089–100.

Chapter 4
Imaging Techniques in Staging and Early Phases

Cristina Nanni

Introduction

The role of imaging in the work-up of patients with multiple myeloma (MM) is aimed to allow the recognition of both the effects of myeloma cells on the skeletal system and the eventual presence of extramedullary disease.

In patients affected by multiple myeloma (MM), bone damage in terms of presence of lytic lesions can be detected in more than 80% of cases at diagnosis and represents one of the criteria (C.R.A.B.) necessary to define a symptomatic or active disease requiring an immediate therapeutic approach [1–3]. Although conventional radiography has historically been the standard of care for many years, in 2014, the IMWG updated the definition of MM, by incorporating novel criteria in the definition of MM defining bone lesions, including not only the presence of at least one lytic lesion detected by skel-

C. Nanni (✉)
Nuclear Medicine, AOU S Orsola-Malpighi, Bologna, Italy
e-mail: cristina.nanni@aosp.bo.it

E. Zamagni (ed.), *Management of Bone Disease and Kidney Failure in Multiple Myeloma*,
https://doi.org/10.1007/978-3-030-63662-3_4

etal radiography but also one focal lesion at CT, FDG-PET/CT, or MRI [4].

Beside a role in recognizing an active MM, the presence of bone disease is the major cause of morbidity and needs to be detected for preventing fractures and spine compression.

Whole Body X-Ray

The whole-body X-ray has been widely used for the identification of osteolytic lesions and has been the standard of care for many years. However, it has several limitations. First drawback is its low sensitivity. To become apparent, in fact, a lytic lesion must present more than 30% loss of trabecular bone, meaning that its detection occurs in a late phase. Furthermore, there are anatomically complicated sites to assess such as the spine and pelvis where the sensitivity can be even lower.

Being a purely morphological imaging, the whole-body X-ray is not appropriate to assess therapy efficacy since most lytic lesions remain unchanged even in complete responder patients.

Last but not least there is an issue regarding specificity that is reduced for the differential diagnosis of myeloma-related fracture and benign fracture.

The MM findings seen on conventional radiographs are lytic lesions with endosteal scalloping, mottled areas of multiple small lesions, diffuse osteopenia, and neoplastic or osteoporotic fractures. One interesting consideration is that MM lesions, unlike most bone metastases, do not exhibit a sclerotic halo owing to the decrease in osteoblastic activity [5, 6].

Whole Body Low-Dose CT

To overcome the limitations of whole-body X-ray, whole-body low-dose CT (WBLDCT) has been proposed in the clinical practice and was proved to be a more sensitive method for detecting even tiny focal lytic lesions. Although low dosage provided in case of MM study as compared to standard diagnostic CT comes at the cost of reduced image quality overall, the study of the skeleton is not significantly impaired due to the intrinsic contrast between high-density mineralized bone and soft-tissue density osteolytic lesions.

Beside sensitivity, whole-body LDCT presents other advantages over whole-body X-ray such as the superiority in estimating fracture risk and bone instability, a really reduced duration of the examination, the production of higher-quality 3D high-resolution images for planning biopsies and therapeutic interventions, and demonstration of unsuspected manifestations of myeloma in the lungs and kidneys. Major disadvantage remains lack of specificity for the differential diagnosis between malignant and osteoporotic fractures. Furthermore, although exposure to radiation is much lower as compared to standard CT, it remains higher than whole-body X-ray: mean dose is approximately 2.8–3.6 mSv as compared to 1.2 mSv for whole-body X-ray.

The WBLDCT exam should be performed on a multidetector scanner with at least 16 detector rows, allowing for very short scanning times and acquisition of thin slices. Field of view should cover from the cranial vault to at least the proximal metaphysis of the tibia. It was suggested to use a 120 kV voltage and a time-current product between 40 and 50 mAs, but other approaches are possible. A narrow collimation protocol with iterative reconstruction algorithms are preferable because they provide a substantial reduction of both image noise and artifacts. "Bone" algorithm can also be used for image post-processing, and slice thickness from 2 to 3 mm is optimal.

The soft tissue reconstruction algorithm images are also useful for assessment of paramedullary and extramedullary soft tissue masses as well as of focal and diffuse hyperdense myeloma deposits in the medullary cavities of the long bones.

Sagittal and coronal multiplanar reformations can be easily generated. In particular, sagittal cuts are helpful to provide an overview on the entire spine to assess disease extent and presence of osteoporosis and risk of fractures and to make a differential diagnosis between malignancy and benign findings (e.g., Schmorl nodules vs lytic lesions).

Another important point is that WBLDCT is one of the FDG PET/CT image sets and can be reconstructed according to specific parameters to optimize the slice thickness and post-filtering. In the end, in one exam it is possible to provide to the clinician functional and morphological data, particularly useful at staging.

The CT findings of MM are essentially the same as the skeletal survey findings: lytic lesions, diffuse osteopenia, endosteal scalloping, neoplastic and osteoporotic fractures, cortical disruption, and extraosseous involvement. Moreover, bone marrow infiltration, especially in the long bones, may appear as hyperattenuating lesions in the soft-tissue window only, without significant osteolysis.

As skeletal survey, WBLDCT is considered not appropriate to assess therapy efficacy since most lytic lesions remain unchanged even in complete responder patients.

Finally, it is important to realize that WBLD CT has a good positive predictive value (94.1%) when osteolytic bone lesions are detected, confirming the diagnosis of MM, but it has a much weaker negative predictive value (58.8%). Therefore, if there are no bone lesions at WBLD CT, then a follow-up investigation with WB MRI (or PET/CT if WB MRI is not available) should be performed [6–9].

MRI

In the last two decades, MRI has emerged as a valuable imaging modality because of its ability to directly visualize bone marrow infiltration much earlier than myeloma-related bone destruction, with no radiation exposure [10], outperforming WBXR and whole-body CT. Moreover, since it is really sensitive for diffuse bone marrow infiltration and small volume disease [11–16], nowadays MRI is considered the imaging gold-standard method for the detection of bone marrow involvement in MM [10] especially at staging. One of the major advantages of MRI is the ability to discriminate between myelomatous and normal bone marrow, allowing to differentiate myeloma from osteoporotic fractures in more than 90% of the cases [17, 18] and to localize spinal cord and nerve root compression [10, 19], as well as the presence of soft tissue extension and/or extramedullary plasmacytomas [20–22].

Several MRI techniques have been developed for the assessment of bone marrow involvement in hematological malignancies [23]. T1-weighted (T1-w) sequences are the best to evaluate bone marrow because they are extremely accurate for the depiction of lipids within the adipocytes [24].

On the other side, T2-weighted (T2-w) sequences are of limited value in evaluating the bone marrow itself [60] because they provide less apparent contrast between yellow and red marrow and have a limited sensitivity for the detection of marrow lesions. However, axial and sagittal T2-w images of the spine are of great importance when suspecting a neurological complication.

Fat-suppression sequences can be added to the standard T1 and T2 and play a crucial role in bone marrow imaging increasing sensitivity for the detection of cellular lesions in the bone marrow [25].

Gadolinium-enhanced MRI can also be used to highlight with high sensitivity the MM-related neoangiogenesis that can be distinguished from red marrow (highly vascularized as well), through the use of fat saturated T1-w.

In addition to this, in the last years, DWI-MRI diffusion weighted sequences (segmental or whole body) have been introduced in the clinical practice, despite are not widely used yet. DW-MRI produces images where the contrast between tissues is based on differences in the motion of water at a cellular level and can provide a semiquantitative parameter related to the probability of malignancy (ADC, apparent diffusion coefficient).

The excellent image contrast between normal and diseased marrow on DW MRI results in superior lesion conspicuity compared to conventional STIR and contrast-enhanced MRI sequences [26, 27]. Furthermore, the ADC value of myeloma infiltrated marrow is significantly different to normal adult marrow with little overlap [28, 29].

Owing to the significant advances in MRI software and hardware, the study of the entire body using MRI is by now a well-established reality. The fact that predilection sites of marrow involvement in MM are not limited to the axial skeleton (i.e., spine and pelvis) may already be considered by itself a valuable reason to justify a whole-body approach for an adequate assessment of the disease, despite peripheral focal lesions only are present in a minor percentage of patients (approximately 10%). Therefore, relatively recently the International Myeloma Working Group established that whole-body MRI represents the standard of reference for the detection of bone marrow involvement in MM, while MRI of the spine and pelvis only can be used in situations where whole-body coverage is not available [30].

Five MRI patterns of marrow involvement have been recognized in multiple myeloma: (1) a focal pattern that consists of localized areas of myeloma cell infiltration 5 mm or greater in diameter, (2) a diffuse pattern characterized by almost complete replacement of normal marrow by myeloma cells, (3) a combined diffuse and focal pattern, (4) a normal bone marrow pattern, and (5) a variegated or "salt and pepper" pattern with uncountable small bone marrow focal lesions.

These patterns need to be recognized at staging because they classify patients into different prognostic groups. For example, the presence of more than one focal lesion on MRI is an independent adverse prognostic factor for progression to active disease. More than 7 focal lesions or a diffuse MRI pattern is related, as well, to a worse prognosis in terms of overall survival.

FDG PET/CT

Fluorodeoxyglucose-F18 18F FDG-PET/CT (positron emission tomography/computed tomography) is a dual technique that blends the ability to identify bone destruction and lytic lesions (LDCT) with the assessment of tumor burden and disease activity (PET), in different areas of the bone marrow (BM), cortical bone, but also soft tissues and organs.

Objective and practical advantages of this technique are the extended field of view (including the skull, ribs, upper limbs, femurs, pelvis, and spine), the absence of possible collateral effects or adverse reactions, the possibility to perform the procedure in patients with renal failure, the fast image acquisition time with 3D tomographs (this is important for patients with fractures, bone pain, or vertebral collapses) and with a standardized procedure, a free decubitus comfortable for patients with severe pain, the possibility to evaluate soft tissues and organs at the same time, the possibility to semi-quantify the disease activity by means of SUV max, the possibility to describe morphological appearances of bones at low-dose CT, and no restrictions in case of metallic bone implants.

It is common knowledge that FDG PET/CT is an appropriate tool to stage MM patients: there is a rich literature proving its added value in terms of number of detection of focal lesions even in a "premorphological" phase, infiltration of the bone marrow, and presence of extramedullary disease [31, 32].

The biological principle at the basis of this procedure is that FDG accumulation in tissue is proportional to the amount of glucose utilization and, therefore, to cell proliferation and malignancy. Increased consumption of glucose is a characteristic of most cancers (including Multiple Myeloma) and is in part related to overexpression of the GLUT-1 glucose transporters and increased hexokinase activity. This increased tracer uptake occurs before myelomatous conglomerates produce a detectable bone damage, making FDG PET/CT an optimal and sensitive tool to stage the disease and defining an active myeloma [33].

It must be reminded, however, that approximately 10% of active myelomas at staging present with a false-negative FDG PET/CT scan because of a transitional lack of hexokinase activity (which eventually can be overexpressed).

Sometimes these patients have several lytic lesions at staging not showing FDG uptake at all [33].

Interestingly, a so-called "false-negative" FDG PET/CT at staging still retains a strong prognostic value, identifying patients with a more favorable progression-free and overall survival [34].

It has been clearly demonstrated that the characteristics of PET involvement at diagnosis represent an important prognostic factor. The number of FLs (>3), the SUVmax value (>4.2 or Deauville Score ≥ 4), diffuse and significant increase in the bone marrow uptake (Deauville Score ≥ 4), and the presence of EMD are significantly related to shorter PFS and OS, retaining independent prognostic relevance. This is the reason why FDG PET/CT is suggested in the initial work-up of the disease by the IMWG recommendations. Furthermore, a basal scan is fundamental for subsequent PET therapy assessment [35–37].

At staging, some advices for correctly interpreting the scan are necessary and are related to the biology of the disease and to the aspecificity of the mechanism of tracer uptake that is accumulated not only by cancer cells but also by inflammatory cells. Most common problems at staging are the presence of MM-related anemia that may result in a significant increase in BM tracer uptake causing a hot background especially in the spine; early PET-positive MM lesions may not correspond to an osteolytic area and may be difficult to call especially if small; recent fractures may appear falsely positive; bone metallic implants may cause significant artefacts on CT and PET images and may be a site of infection with a consequent nonspecific FDG uptake; "salt and pepper" pattern may not be detectable (lesions are too small).

Recently, different standard interpretation criteria have been proposed. Mesguich et al. [38] proposed some indications to interpret MM FDG-PET/CT in staging, during and after therapy, but these remain general suggestions. Other groups proposed SUV-derived parameters such as total lesion glycolysis (TLG) and metabolic tumor volume (MTV) [39] to assess the active disease burden at baseline and its variation (delta) as a consequence of therapy. However, a standard and widely accepted software program to harmonize MTV or TLG measure in clinical practice is still lacking. Furthermore, none of the proposed criteria have been clinically validated.

In the last years, visual descriptive criteria (Italian Myeloma criteria for Pet Use: IMPeTUs) were proposed to standardize FDG PET/CT evaluation in MM patients [40]. These include the visual interpretation of images to quantify FDG uptake using the five points scale of Deauville score (DS) proposed for interim and final FDG PET in lymphoma [41], in association with a morphological and anatomical aspect of FDG distribution such as the bone marrow non-focal uptake, focal bone lesions (site, number and uptake), and paramedullary or extramedullary lesions.

This way of standardizing PET reading, according to described criteria, and procedure according to published guidelines [42] makes FDG PET/CT a reproducible tool providing functional and morphological data at the same time at staging.

References

1. Terpos E, Politou M, Rahemtulla A. New insights into the pathophysiology and management of bone disease in multiple myeloma. Br J Haematol. 2003;123:758Y769.
2. Lecouvet FE, Malghem J, Michaux L, et al. Skeletal survey in advanced multiple myeloma: radiographic versus MR imaging survey. Br J Haematol. 1999;106:35Y39.
3. Umeda M, Adachi Y, Tomiyama J, et al. Bone lesions in elderly multiple myeloma. Nippon Ronen Igakkai Zasshi. 2002;39:631Y638.
4. Rajkumar SV, Dimopoulos MA, Palumbo A, et al. International myeloma working group updated criteria for the diagnosis of multiple myeloma. Lancet Oncol. 2014;15:e538–48.
5. Dimopoulos M, Terpos E, Comenzo RL, et al. International myeloma working group consensus statement and guidelines regarding the current role of imaging techniques in the

diagnosis and monitoring of multiple myeloma. Leukemia. 2009;23:1545–56.
6. Terpos E, Moulopoulos LA, Dimopoulos MA. Advances in imaging and the management of myeloma bone disease. J Clin Oncol. 2011;29:1907–15.
7. Pianko MJ, Terpos E, Roodman GD, et al. Whole-body low-dose computed tomography and advanced imaging techniques for multiple myeloma bone disease. Clin Cancer Res. 2014;20:5888–97.
8. Ippolito D, Besostri V, Bonaffini PA, et al. Diagnostic value of whole- body low-dose computed tomography (WBLDCT) in bone lesions detection in patients with multiple myeloma (MM). Eur J Radiol. 2013;82:2322–7.
9. Horger M, Claussen CD, Bross-Bach U, et al. Whole-body low-dose multidetector row-CT in the diagnosis of multiple myeloma: an alternative to conventional radiography. Eur J Radiol. 2005;54:289–97.
10. Dimopoulos MA, Hillengass J, Usmani S, Zamagni E, Lentzsch S, Davies FE, Raje N, Sezer O, Zweegman S, Shah J, et al. Role of magnetic resonance imaging in the management of patients with multiple myeloma: a consensus statement. J Clin Oncol. 2015;33:657–64.
11. Zamagni E, Nanni C, Patriarca F, et al. A prospective comparison of 18F-fluorodeoxyglucose positron emission tomography-computed tomography, magnetic resonance imaging and whole body planar radiographs in the assessment of bone disease in newly diagnosed multiple myeloma. Haematologica. 2007;92:50–5.
12. Waheed S, Mitchell A, Usmani S, et al. Standard and novel imaging methods for multiple myeloma: correlates with prognostic laboratory variables including gene expression profiling data. Haematologica. 2013;98:71–8.
13. Breyer RJ III, Mulligan ME, Smith SE, Line BR, Badros AZ. Comparison of imaging with FDG PET/CT with other imaging modalities in myeloma. Skelet Radiol. 2006;35:632–40.
14. Spinnato P, Bazzocchi A, Brioli A, Nanni C, Zamagni E, Albisinni U, et al. Contrast enhanced MRI and (1)(8)F-FDG PET-CT in the assessment of multiple myeloma: a comparison of results in different phases of the disease. Eur J Radiol. 2012;81:4013–8.
15. Shortt CP, Gleeson TG, Breen KA, et al. Whole-body MRI versus PET in assessment of multiple myeloma disease activity. AJR Am J Roentgenol. 2009;192:980–6.

16. Moreau P, Attal M, Caillot D, et al. Prospective evaluation of magnetic resonance imaging and [18F] fluorodeoxyglucose positron emission tomography-computed tomography at diagnosis and before maintenance therapy in symptomatic patients with multiple myeloma included in the IFM/DFCI 2009 trial: results of the IMAJEM study. J Clin Oncol. 2017;35(25):2911–8.
17. Moulopoulos LA, Dimopoulos MA. Magnetic resonance imaging of the bone marrow in hematologic malignancies. Blood. 1997;90:2127–47.
18. Baur A, Stabler A, Bruning R, et al. Diffusion-weighted MR imaging of bone marrow: differentiation of benign versus pathologic compression fractures. Radiology. 1998;207:349–56. https://doi.org/10.1148/radiology.207.2.9577479.
19. Joffe J, Williams MP, Cherryman GR, Gore M, McElwain TJ, Selby P. Magnetic resonance imaging in myeloma. Lancet. 1998;21:1162–3.
20. Moulopoulos LA, Dimopoulos MA, Weber D, et al. Magnetic resonance imaging in the staging of solitary plasmacytoma of bone. J Clin Oncol. 1993;11:1311–5. https://doi.org/10.1200/JCO.1993.11.7.1311.
21. Dimopoulos MA, Moulopoulos LA, Maniatis A, et al. Solitary plasmacytoma of bone and asymptomatic multiple myeloma. Blood. 2000;96:2037–44.
22. Varettoni M, Corso A, Pica G, et al. Incidence, presenting features and outcome of extramedullary disease in multiple myeloma: a longitudinal study on 1003 consecutive patients. Ann Oncol. 2010;21:325–30.
23. Klein B, Tarte K, Jourdan M, Mathouk K, Moreaux J, Jourdan E, Legouffe E, De Vos J, Rossi JF. Survival and proliferation factors of normal and malignant plasma cells. Int J Hematol. 2003;78:106–13.
24. Reiser MF, Hricak H, Knauth M. Magnetic resonance imaging of the bone marrow. In: Baur-Melnyk A, editor. Medical radiology, diagnostic imaging. Berlin: Springer; 2013.
25. Vande Berg BC, Malghem J, Lecouvet FE, et al. Magnetic resonance imaging of normal bone marrow. Eur Radiol. 1998;8:1327–34.
26. Pearce T, Philip S, Brown J, Koh DM, Burn PR. Bone metastases from prostate, breast and multiple myeloma: differences in lesion conspicuity at short-tau inversion recovery and diffusion-weighted MRI. Br J Radiol. 2012;85(1016):1102–6.

27. Dutoit JC, Vanderkerken MA, Anthonissen J, Dochy F, Verstraete KL. The diagnostic value of SE MRI and DWI of the spine in patients with monoclonal gammopathy of undetermined significance, smouldering myeloma and multiple myeloma. Eur Radiol. 2014;24(11):2754–65.
28. Hillengass J, Bäuerle T, Bartl R, et al. Diffusion-weighted imaging for non-invasive and quantitative monitoring of bone marrow infiltration in patients with monoclonal plasma cell disease: a comparative study with histology. Br J Haematol. 2011;153(6):721–8.
29. Messiou C, Collins DJ, Morgan VA, Desouza NM. Optimising diffusion weighted MRI for imaging metastatic and myeloma bone disease and assessing reproducibility. Eur Radiol. 2011;21(8):1713–8.
30. Terpos E, Dimopoulos MA. Myeloma bone disease: pathophysiology and management. Ann Oncol. 2015;16:1223–31.
31. Zamagni E, Nanni C, Patriarca F, Englaro E, Castellucci P, Geatti O, Tosi P, Tacchetti P, Cangini D, Perrone G, Ceccolini M, Brioli A, Buttignol S, Fanin R, Salizzoni E, Baccarani M, Fanti S, Cavo M. A prospective comparison of 18F-fluorodeoxyglucose positron emission tomography-computed tomography, magnetic resonance imaging and whole-body planar radiographs in the assessment of bone disease in newly diagnosed multiple myeloma. Haematologica. 2007;92(1):50–5.
32. Nanni C, Zamagni E, Farsad M, Castellucci P, Tosi P, Cangini D, Salizzoni E, Canini R, Cavo M, Fanti S. Role of 18F-FDG PET/CT in the assessment of bone involvement in newly diagnosed multiple myeloma: preliminary results. Eur J Nucl Med Mol Imaging. 2006;33(5):525–31. Epub 2006 Feb 2
33. Rasche L, Angtuaco E, McDonald JE, Buros A, Stein C, Pawlyn C, Thanendrarajan S, Schinke C, Samant R, Yaccoby S, Walker BA, Epstein J, Zangari M, van Rhee F, Meissner T, Goldschmidt H, Hemminki K, Houlston R, Barlogie B, Davies FE, Morgan GJ, Weinhold N. Low expression of hexokinase-2 is associated with false-negative FDG-positron emission tomography in multiple myeloma. Blood. 2017;130(1):30–4. https://doi.org/10.1182/blood-2017-03-774422. Epub 2017 Apr 21
34. Abe Y, Ikeda S, Kitadate A, Narita K, Kobayashi H, Miura D, Takeuchi M, O'uchi E, O'uchi T, Matsue K. Low hexokinase-2 expression-associated false-negative 18F-FDG PET/CT as a potential prognostic predictor in patients with multiple

myeloma. Eur J Nucl Med Mol Imaging. 2019;46(6):1345–50. https://doi.org/10.1007/s00259-019-04312-9. Epub 2019 Mar 22

35. Bartel TB, Haessler J, Brown TL, Shaughnessy JD Jr, van Rhee F, Anaissie E, Alpe T, Angtuaco E, Walker R, Epstein J, Crowley J, Barlogie B. F18-fluorodeoxyglucose positron emission tomography in the context of other imaging techniques and prognostic factors in multiple myeloma. Blood. 2009;114(10):2068–76. https://doi.org/10.1182/blood-2009-03-213280. Epub 2009 May 14
36. Zamagni E, Patriarca F Nanni C, Zannetti B, Englaro E, Pezzi A, Tacchetti P, Buttignol S, Perrone G, Brioli A, Pantani L, Terragna C, Carobolante F, Baccarani M, Fanin R, Fanti S, Cavo M. Prognostic relevance of 18-F FDG PET/CT in newly diagnosed multiple myeloma patients treated with up-front autologous transplantation. Blood. 2011;118(23):5989–95. https://doi.org/10.1182/blood-2011-06-361386. Epub 2011 Sep 6. Erratum in: Blood. 2012 Sep 13;120(11):2349.
37. Moreau P, Attal M, Caillot D, Macro M, Karlin L, Garderet L, Facon T, Benboubker L, Escoffre-Barbe M, Stoppa AM, Laribi K, Hulin C, Perrot A, Marit G, Eveillard JR, Caillon F, Bodet-Milin C, Pegourie B, Dorvaux V, Chaleteix C, Anderson K, Richardson P, Munshi NC, Avet-Loiseau H, Gaultier A, Nguyen JM, Dupas B, Frampas E, Kraeber-Bodere F. Prospective evaluation of magnetic resonance imaging and [18F]fluorodeoxyglucose positron emission tomography-computed tomography at diagnosis and before maintenance therapy in symptomatic patients with multiple myeloma included in the IFM/DFCI 2009 trial: results of the IMAJEM Study. J Clin Oncol. 2017;35(25):2911–8. https://doi.org/10.1200/JCO.2017.72.2975. Epub 2017 Jul 7.
38. Mesguich C, Fardanesh R, Tanenbaum L, Chari A, Jagannath S, Kostakoglu L. State of the art imaging of multiple myeloma: comparative review of FDG PET/CT imaging in various clinical settings. Eur J Radiol. 2014;83(12):2203–23. https://doi.org/10.1016/j.ejrad.2014.09.012. Epub 2014 Sep 28
39. McDonald JE, Kessler MM, Gardner MW, Buros AF, Ntambi JA, Waheed S, van Rhee F, Zangari M, Heuck CJ, Petty N, Schinke C, Thanendrarajan S, Mitchell A, Hoering A, Barlogie B, Morgan GJ, Davies FE. Assessment of total lesion glycolysis by 18F FDG PET/CT significantly improves prognostic value of GEP and ISS in myeloma. Clin Cancer Res. 2017;23(8):1981–7. https://doi.org/10.1158/1078-0432.CCR-16-0235. Epub 2016 Oct 3

40. Nanni C, Versari A, Chauvie S, Bertone E, Bianchi A, Rensi M, Bellò M, Gallamini A, Patriarca F, Gay F, Gamberi B, Ghedini P, Cavo M, Fanti S, Zamagni E. Interpretation criteria for FDG PET/CT in multiple myeloma (IMPeTUs): final results. IMPeTUs (Italian myeloma criteria for PET USe). Eur J Nucl Med Mol Imaging. 2018;45(5):712–9. https://doi.org/10.1007/s00259-017-3909-8. Epub 2017 Dec 21
41. Itti E, Meignan M, Berriolo-Riedinger A, Biggi A, Cashen AF, Véra P, Tilly H, Siegel BA, Gallamini A, Casasnovas RO, Haioun C. An international confirmatory study of the prognostic value of early PET/CT in diffuse large B-cell lymphoma: comparison between Deauville criteria and ΔSUVmax. Eur J Nucl Med Mol Imaging. 2013;40(9):1312–20. https://doi.org/10.1007/s00259-013-2435-6. Epub 2013 May 7
42. Boellaard R, Delgado-Bolton R, Oyen WJG, Giammarile F, Tatsch K, Eschner W, Verzijlbergen FJ, Barrington SF, Pike LC, Weber WA, Stroobants S, Delbeke D, Donohoe KJ, Holbrook S, Graham MM, Testanera G, Hoekstra OS, Zijlstra J, Visser E, Hoekstra CJ, Pruim J, Willemsen A, Arends B, Kotzerke J, Bockisch A, Beyer T, Chiti A, Krause BJ. FDG PET/CT: EANM procedure guidelines for tumour imaging: version 2.0. Eur J Nucl Med Mol Imaging. 2015;42:328–54.

Chapter 5
Imaging Techniques for Response Assessment and Follow-Up

Leo Rasche, Anke Heidemeier, Stefan Delorme, and Niels Weinhold

L. Rasche (✉)
Department of Internal Medicine 2, University Hospital of Würzburg, Würzburg, Germany

Mildred Scheel Early Career Center (MSNZ), University Hospital of Würzburg, Würzburg, Germany

Myeloma Center, University of Arkansas for Medical Sciences, Little Rock, AR, USA
e-mail: Rasche_L@ukw.de

A. Heidemeier
Department of Radiology, University Hospital of Würzburg, Würzburg, Germany

S. Delorme
Department of Radiology, German Cancer Research Center, Heidelberg, Germany

N. Weinhold
Myeloma Center, University of Arkansas for Medical Sciences, Little Rock, AR, USA

Department of Internal Medicine V, University Hospital of Heidelberg, Heidelberg, Germany

E. Zamagni (ed.), *Management of Bone Disease and Kidney Failure in Multiple Myeloma*,
https://doi.org/10.1007/978-3-030-63662-3_5

Introduction

In multiple myeloma (MM), the disease distribution within the bone marrow (BM) space is usually heterogeneous with the spine, pelvis, and sternum being the most involved skeletal regions [1]. Up to 80% of newly diagnosed MM patients (NDMM) present with focal lesions (FLs) which are discrete MM cell accumulations that may occur at any site in the BM-containing skeletal system (Fig. 5.1). In the majority of patients, these FLs are superimposed on diffusively growing

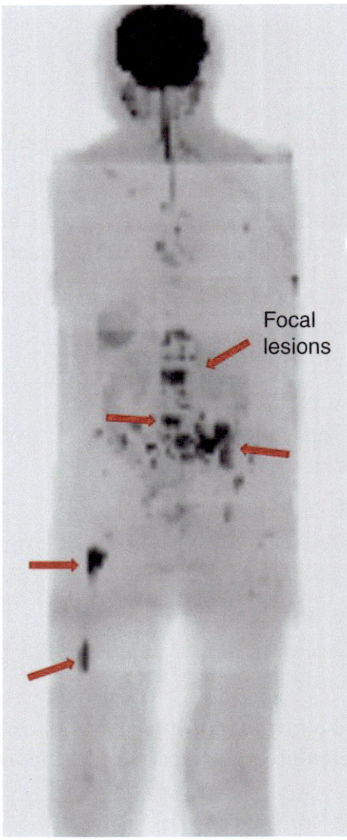

FIGURE 5.1 Diffusion-weighted MRI of relapse refractory myeloma patient presenting with multiple large focal lesions in the axial and appendicular skeleton

MM cells [2]. In contrast, macrofocal MM, which is seen in 6% of NDMM patients, is characterized by the presence of osteolytic FLs without intervening diffuse BM infiltration [3, 4]. Solitary plasmacytoma of the bone (SPB) with or without minimal BM infiltration is another example for the heterogeneous disease distribution in MM and seen in 5% of NDMM patients [5].

The number and location of FLs has been linked to poor prognosis [2, 6–8]. To shed light on the mechanism underlying the prognostic impact of FLs, we performed next-generation sequencing of BM samples collected from multiple regions and showed that the genomic makeup of clones from FLs often differs from that found in the iliac crest, the routine origin of BM specimens [9]. In a relevant number of patients, high-risk clones characterized by adverse genomic features, such as biallelic *TP53* events, were restricted to FLs and not detectable at the iliac crest, highlighting that BM specimens from a single site are not always representative for the entire BM cavity. This type of intratumor heterogeneity was mainly seen in patients with large FLs (diameter > 2.5 cm). Using the size of FLs as surrogate marker for spatial genomic heterogeneity, we recently identified the presence of multiple large focal lesions as an adverse prognostic factor in NDMM [10]. Based on our observations, we hypothesized that multiple large FLs reflect an advanced stage of tumor evolution associated with an increased level of spatial genomic heterogeneity and clonal diversity. As a result, there is a higher probability for the presence of treatment-resistant tumor subclones that are spatially separated in these patients. *It is critical to note that spatial clonal heterogeneity could potentially lead to spatial differences in response to anti-MM therapy*. Indeed, we recently noted mixed radiological response of FLs with some of them progressing in size whereas others resolved during therapy [11, 12]. Unique subclones dominate in resistant lesions, and multiple spatially separated clones can survive extensive treatment in patients who achieve CR and are classified as minimal residual disease (MRD) negative based on a sample from the iliac crest [11]. Similarly, extramedullary disease (EMD) has been reported to frequently progress without significant BM involvement [13, 14]. These observations are in line with spatially separated clones that respond differently to treatment. Since resistant clones frequently evolve in FLs, we suggest that medical imaging is the key to tackle the limitations of response assessments that are based on conventional criteria and a single BM sample from the iliac crest.

In 2006, the International Myeloma Working Group (IMWG) did not yet consider imaging for response assessment [15].Only for situations suspicious for progressive disease, the authors stated "whatever additional testing is required to confirm myeloma relatedness is strongly encouraged. This may include magnetic resonance imaging (MRI), computed tomography (CT) and/or fluoro-18-deoxyglucose (FDG)/positron emission tomography (PET) imaging." Yet, based on the idea that non-secretory and extramedullary disease is not easily accessible by conventional response evaluation and MRD diagnostics, respectively, the IMWG released a position paper in 2016, in which the authors also suggested imaging as an additional element of response evaluation (Table 5.1) [16]. Basically, the deepest level of response was allocated to patients in complete remission (CR) according to the standard criteria and displaying MRD negative BM by next-generation flow or sequencing and no evidence of active disease on imaging. Partial remission (PR) was defined as ≥50% reduction of serum M-protein plus reduction in 24 h urinary M-protein by ≥90% or to <200 mg per 24 h and, if present at baseline, a ≥ 50% reduction in the size (sum of perpendicular diameters, SPD) of soft tissue plasmacytomas. Appearance of a new lesion(s), ≥50% increase from nadir in SPD of >1 lesion, or ≥ 50% increase in the longest diameter of a previous lesion >1 cm in short axis was defined as progressive disease. Of note, the authors recommended the CT part of the PET-CT, or MRI scans, or dedicated CT scans for plasmacytoma measurement. The authors did not embark on the use of functional imaging such as FDG PET-CT or diffusion-weighted MRI (DW-MRI) for response evaluation. A recent IMWG consensus paper on the use of imaging in plasma cell disorders addresses imaging modalities in more detail [17], and we will discuss recommendations of this paper regarding response evaluation in our article.

Table 5.1 IMWG criteria for response assessment including criteria for minimal residual disease

	Response criteria
IMWG MRD criteria (requires a complete response as defined below)	
Sustained MRD-negative	MRD negativity in the marrow (NGF or NGS, or both) and by imaging as defined below, confirmed minimum of 1 year apart. Subsequent evaluations can be used to further specify the duration of negativity (eg, MRD-negative at 5 years)
Flow MRD-negative	The absence of phenotypically aberrant clonal plasma cells by NGF on bone marrow aspirates using the EuroFlow standard operation procedure for MRD detection in multiple myeloma (or validated equivalent method) with a minimum sensitivity of 1 in 10 nucleated 5 cells or higher
Sequencing MRD-negative	The absence of clonal plasma cells by NGS on bone marrow aspirate in which the presence of a clone is defined as less than two identical sequencing reads obtained after DNA sequencing of bone marrow aspirates using the LymphoSIGHT platform (or validated equivalent method) with a minimum sensitivity of 1 in 105 nucleated cells or higher
Imaging plus MRD-negative	MRD negativity as defined by NGF or NGS plus disappearance of every area of increased tracer uptake found at baseline or a preceding PET/CT or decrease to less mediastinal blood pool SUV or decrease to less than that of surrounding normal tissue
Standard IMWG responsecriteria	
Stringent completeresponse	Complete response as defined below plus normal FLC ratio and the absence of clonal cells in bone marrow biopsy by immunohistochemistry (κ/λ ratio ≤4:1 or ≥1:2 for κ and λ patients, respectively, after counting ≥100 plasma cells)
Completeresponse	Negative immunofixation on the serum and urine and disappearance of any soft tissue plasmacytomas and <5% plasma cells in bone marrow aspirates
Very good partial response	Serum and urine M-protein detectable by immunofixation but not on electrophoresis or ≥90% reduction in serum M-protein plus urine M-protein level <100 mg per 24 h
Partial response	≥50% reduction of serum M-protein plus reduction in 24 h urinary M-protein by ≥90% or to <200 mg per 24 h;
	If the serum and urine M-protein are unmeasurable, a ≥50% decrease in the difference between involved and uninvolved FLC levels is required in place of the M-protein criteria
	If serum and urine M-protein are unmeasurable, and serum-free light assay is also unmeasurable, ≥50% reduction in plasma cells is required in place of M-protein, provided baseline bone marrow plasma-cell percentage was ≥30%. In addition to these criteria, if present at baseline, a ≥50% reduction in the size (SPD) of soft tissue plasmacytomas is also required
Minimal response	≥25% but ≤49% reduction of serum M-protein and reduction in 24-h urine M-protein by 50–89%. In addition to the above listed criteria, if present at baseline, a ≥50% reduction in the size (SPD) of soft tissue plasmacytomas is also required
Stable disease	Not recommended for use as an indicator of response; stability of disease is best described by providing the time-to-progression estimates. Not meeting criteria for complete response, very good partial response, partial response, minimal response, or progressive disease
Progressive disease	Any one or more of the following criteria:
	Increase of 25% from lowest confirmed response value in one or more of the following criteria:
	Serum M-protein (absolute increase must be ≥0·5 g/dL);

TABLE 5.1 (continued)

	Serum M-protein increase ≥1 g/dL, if the lowest M component was ≥5 g/dL;
	Urine M-protein (absolute increase must be ≥200 mg/24 h);
	In patients without measurable serum and urine M-protein levels, the difference between involved and uninvolved FLC levels (absolute increase must be >10 mg/dL); In patients without measurable serum and urine M-protein levels and without measurable involved FLC levels, bone marrow plasma-cell percentage irrespective of baseline status (absolute increase must be ≥10%);
	Appearance of a new lesion(s), ≥50% increase from nadir in SPD of >1 lesion, or ≥50% increase in the longest diameter of a previous lesion >1 cm in short axis;
	≥50% increase in circulating plasma cells (minimum of 200 cells per µL) if this is the only measure of disease
Clinical relapse	Clinical relapse requires one or more of the following criteria:
	Direct indicators of increasing disease and/or end organ dysfunction (CRAB features) related to the underlying clonal plasma-cell proliferative disorder. It is not used in calculation of time to progression or progression-free survival but is listed as something that can be reported optionally or for use in clinical practice;
	Development of new soft tissue plasmacytomas or bone lesions (osteoporotic fractures do not constitute progression);
	Definite increase in the size of existing plasmacytomas or bone lesions. A definite increase is defined as a 50% (and ≥ 1 cm) increase as measured serially by the SPD of the measurable lesion;
	Hypercalcaemia (>11 mg/dL);
	Decrease in haemoglobin of ≥2 g/dL not related to therapy or other non-myeloma-related conditions;
	Rise in serum creatinine by 2 mg/dL or more from the start of the therapy and attributable to myeloma;
	Hyperviscosity related to serum paraprotein
Relapse from complete response (to be used only if the end point is disease-free survival)	Any one or more of the following criteria:
	Reappearance of serum or urine M-protein by immunofixation or electrophoresis;
	Development of ≥5% plasma cells in the bone marrow;
	Appearance of any other sign of progression (ie, new plasmacytoma, lytic bone lesion, or hypercalcaemia see above)
Relapse from MRD negative (to be used only if the end point is disease-free survival)	Any one or more of the following criteria:
	Loss of MRD negative state (evidence of clonal plasma cells on NGF or NGS, or positive imaging study for recurrence of myeloma);
	Reappearance of serum or urine M-protein by immunofixation or electrophoresis;
	Development of ≥5% clonal plasma cells in the bone marrow;
	Appearance of any other sign of progression (ie, new plasmacytoma, lytic bone lesion, or hypercalcaemia)

(Adopted from Kumar et al. [16]. Imaging related categories are highlighted in light blue)

Scope of This Article

In this article, we are aiming to provide the reader with a comprehensive overview of the current status of imaging for response assessment in MM by addressing the following questions:

1. *Which techniques should be used for imaging-based response evaluation?* We summarize the literature on response evaluation by anatomical and functional imaging

modalities. We discuss hexokinase-2 (HK2) expression in plasma cells as a confounder of FDG PET-CT scans and present recent data for alternative PET tracers for MM such as L-methyl-[11C]-methionine.

2. *Which is the optimal time point for imaging during follow-up?* We discuss studies that used imaging at fixed time points (e.g., pre-maintenance) versus efforts evaluating individualized time points such as the achievement of CR. In this context, we will also present recent studies which combined MRD assessment with imaging.
3. *How specific and sensitive is imaging in detecting residual disease, and how far are we with standardizing image acquisition and interpretation?* We will discuss the issue of limited sensitivity, specificity, standardization, and experience in terms of medical imaging for response evaluation.
4. *Can imaging already guide therapy decision-making?* In this section, we discuss how medical imaging could alter therapy.

Which Technique Should Be Used for Imaging-Based Response Evaluation?

It is important to discriminate between axial (pelvis, spine, and skull) and whole-body (axial + appendicular skeleton) imaging. Of note, in ~10% of NDMM patients, FLs can only be found in the appendicular skeleton [18], and these FLs have recently been linked to poor prognosis [8], highlighting whole-body imaging to be necessary for initial and follow-up investigations of MM patients. It is also important to distinguish between two major imaging classes: anatomic and functional imaging:

Anatomic Imaging

CT and morphologic MRI are examples for anatomic imaging and detect phenotypic alterations in tissues that are not necessarily associated with active malignant disease [19]. Using CT only, it is difficult to discriminate between inactive, successfully treated lesions and treatment-resistant active lesions [20].The same holds true for conventional MRI. Discrete changes may help in this situation, e.g., a lesion with a sclerotic border on CT is more indicative for a healing bone lesion [21].Similarly, signal decrease on T2-weighted images together with signal recovery on T1-weighted images is considered to be a sign of disease response on MRI [22, 23].Recently, Merz and colleagues reported on a subset of patients, who showed cystic transformation of FLs during treatment characterized by a signal intensity similar to cerebrospinal fluid on T2- and T1-weighted images [24].Although this pattern indicated that the lesion in question had healed, it was nevertheless associated with an overall adverse outcome. However, sensitivity and specificity of these discrete changes on CT or MRI have yet to be clarified, and from our point of view, anatomic imaging alone cannot be recommended for response evaluation.

FDG PET-CT

In contrast to anatomical approaches, functional imaging detects physiologic processes. FDG PET-CT, where an uptake map for FDG is overlaid on an anatomical CT scan, visualizes increased uptake of glucose by tumor cells. Recently, Moreau and colleagues demonstrated that FDG PET-CT is superior to conventional MRI in monitoring response to therapy in 134 patients enrolled in the IMAJEM study [22], although in this whole-body PET/CT study was compared to MRI that was confined to only the axial but not the appendicular skeleton. At diagnosis, MRI and FDG PET-CT scans showed essentially the same number of bone lesions per patient but after therapy signal normalization could mainly be observed on FDG PET-CT (62% versus 11% of patients at the time point pre-maintenance) [22].Normalization of the FDG signal was associated with improved progression-free (PFS) and overall survival (OS) and an independent prognostic factor in multivariate analysis. Of note, the authors defined normalization as uptake less than or equal to liver activity in FLs, BM, and EMD. Likewise, the Little Rock group showed that complete FDG suppression in FLs before first autologous stem cell transplantation (ASCT) was associated with better outcomes in 176 newly diagnosed patients treated with total therapy 3 [25]. Pre-ASCT FDG suppression was even superior to pre-ASCT clinical CR, probably due to the greater prognostic power of FDG suppression encompassing non-secretory myeloma cells. In fact, serological CR or near CR status before ASCT did not affect post-ASCT survival outcomes in this study. The authors used the BM background signal at the lumbar spine as a reference. A positive impact on survival was seen for both gene expression profiling-defined high-risk and low-risk patients. The Bologna group investigated 189 NDMM patients 3 months after the last cycle of first-line treatment with FDG PET-CT to evaluate skeletal response to therapy [26]. Again, achievement of PET negativity significantly impacted PFS and OS, and on multivariate analysis PET normalization was a positive prognostic factor. Patients achieving CR based on the standard IMWG criteria but still had positive PET scans experienced adverse outcomes. The authors used the spleen signal as reference for diffuse BM infiltration, and FLs were defined as circumscribed hypermetabolic uptake greater than the surrounding BM or based on standardized uptake value (SUV)max measurements [26]. Other smaller studies also demonstrated the prognostic value of PET normalization in MM [27–31]. Together, metabolic suppression of MM disease and subsequent normalization of the FDG signal is an independent prognostic factor in NDMM patients.

DW-MRI

The functional imaging modality DW-MRI detects restriction of water diffusion by the lipophilic cell membranes of tumor cell accumulations and can be performed on state-of-the-art

MRI systems supplied by all major vendors [32]. An association between the DW-MRI parameter apparent diffusion coefficient (ADC) and treatment response was demonstrated in several studies [33–36]. More specifically, in patients who responded to treatment, ADC values increased, while non-responders showed stable or decreasing values. To address the question if DW-MRI also improves detection of resistant disease in deep responders, we investigated DWI-MRI data of 186 transplantation-eligible NDMM patients who achieved CR during first-line therapy, and scans were performed as soon as CR had been achieved. We detected residual FLs in 21% of the patients, who had adverse outcome compared to patients without FLs. The poorest outcome was seen in patients with residual FLs and high risk according to the gene expression profiling (GEP)-based GEP70 risk classifier or International Staging System (ISS) III (median PFS of 0.9 years) [11].

FDG PET-CT vs DW-MRI

For follow-up, the IMWG recommends using the same imaging technique that was used at initial diagnosis in order to provide comparability [17]. Which functional imaging technique, however, should be used for disease monitoring? Both, DW-MRI and FDG PET-CT, have their advantages and disadvantages. The disadvantages of DW-MRI are the relatively long scanning time (up to 1 hour) and its limited ability to detect small extramedullary lesions, such as affected lymph nodes. Advantages of this method compared to FDG PET-CT include (1) no pre-scan diet requirements, (2) no exposure to radioactive tracers, and (3) no dependence on the metabolic activity of tumor cells [10]. Especially the dependence on FDG uptake can be major issue of FDG PET-CT. We have recently shown that ~10% of NDMM have high tumor loads according to DW-MRI but are negative according to FDG PET-CT [9]. Low expression of *HK2*, which catalyzes the first step of glycolysis, was strongly associated with false-negativity. Another study confirmed these observations, linking low *HK2* expression to false-negative PET results in 90 patients treated in Japan [37], and in this study, false-negativity was associated with better outcome. Based on the frequent observation of false-negativity at baseline, we expected FDG PET-CT to be less sensitive during follow-up, too. Indeed, in our recent study, only 6% of patients achieving CR had residual FLs on FDG PET-CT scans, while 21% of the patients were positive in DW-MRI [11]. Only six patients presented with FLs that were positive on DW-MRI and FDG PET-CT, and the PFS of patients with FLs, which were only detectable using DW-MRI, was not significantly different from patients with PET-positive FLs.

Several other tracers have been tested to overcome the limitations of FDG PET [38–43]. As an example, L-methyl-[11C]-methionine (MET), which is rapidly taken up into MM cells and incorporated into newly synthesized immunoglobulins, is a promising alternative [39]. Compared to FDG, MET has a higher sensitivity to detect FLs and EMD, but it is important to note that MET PET also depends on the metabolism of tumor cells. On the other hand, despite the limitations linked to quantification of tumor metabolism, PET-CT has major strengths compared to DW-MRI: early detection of "active" residual FLs which do not have increased cellularity compared to their surroundings and the ability to assess (metabolic) disease activity. In our recent study, there were five patients in CR who were DW-MRI negative but presented with FLs in FDG PET-CT, demonstrating that (1) the high dependence on increased cellularity can be a disadvantage of DW-MRI during follow-up studies and (2) a combination of both modalities increases sensitivity for detection of residual disease. We will discuss sensitivity of the two techniques in more detail in the paragraph "Sensitivity, Specificity and Standardization of Imaging for Response Evaluation."

Together, functional imaging is superior to anatomic imaging for response evaluation, and functional parameters such as the SUV and the ADC are strongly associated with conventional response. DW-MRI is the more sensitive method for detection of residual FLs, but FDG PET-CT is a complementary technique which allows for a discrimination between active and inactive residual disease.

Which Is the Optimal Time Point for Imaging During Follow-Up?

Previous studies have investigated functional imaging for response evaluation at various early and late time points. The Little Rock group investigated FDG PET-CT on day 7 of VTD-PACE induction, a multiagent regimen including bortezomib, thalidomide, dexamethasone, and 4 days continuous infusions of cisplatin, doxorubicin, cyclophosphamide, and etoposide. Including 302 patients enrolled in total therapy three trials, the presence of more than three FDG-avid FLs at day 7, which was seen in 36% of patients, was associated with unfavorable outcome, irrespective of the GEP-defined risk status [44]. A French group evaluated the prognostic value of FDG PET-CT after three cycles of lenalidomide, bortezomib, and dexamethasone in patients who were FDG positive at baseline [45]. In multivariate analysis, suppression of FDG uptake, measured as reduction of SUVmax, was a positive prognostic factor. Similar results were reported for another study from Little Rock, which investigated FDG PET-CT prior to first ASCT [25]. Normalization conferred superior overall and event-free survival.

In the prospective Franco-Canadian IMAJEM study, imaging was also performed pre-maintenance after ASCT. 62% of the patients showed suppressed FDG signals before maintenance, and this was associated with improved PFS. Similar results were seen in a small retrospective study investigating PET-CT up to 9 months after ASCT [27].Positive imaging prior to or after allogenic stem cell transplantation was associated with impaired outcome in two independent studies, too [30, 46].

With the aim to better define the optimal time point for follow-up imaging, the Little Rock group investigated longitudinally collected FDG PET-CT scans at day 7 after treatment initiation, post induction, post-ASCT, and prior to maintenance therapy in an extended set of 596 NDMM patients. For all of these time points, patients with no detectable FL at that time point had a significantly superior outcome compared to patients with at least one detectable FL at that time point, irrespective of whether they had an FL at baseline [47]. The authors concluded that serial PET-CT should be integrated into follow-up algorithms and that suppression of focal lesions at any time point constitutes a major therapeutic goal in NDMM.

An alternative approach to fixed time points is imaging at individualized time points such as the achievement of deep responses. Zamagni and colleagues analyzed PET-CT data of patients in CR according to conventional criteria after first-line therapy, and 29% of patients still had positive scans [26]. Median PFS for this group of patients was 44 months and 84 months for PET-positive and PET-negative patients, respectively. Performing a similar study with DW-MRI and PET-CT, we detected residual FLs in 40 of the 168 (24%) patients at the onset of CR, and these lesions were associated with an unfavorable outcome. Combining functional imaging with MRD diagnostics for these patients, we showed that patients with double-positive tests had the worst outcome. On the other hand, patients with negative results in both tests had the best outcome, confirming results of the IMAJEM trial [22] and highlighting that functional imaging complements MRD diagnostics in CR patients. Recently, a study by Alonso and co-workers confirmed these observations [48].

Together, negative imaging scans have been associated with good outcome at multiple time points. The IMWG proposes to perform FDG PET-CT prior to maintenance therapy and recommends follow-up annually in case of detectable residual FL. In our opinion, the time point depends on the aim of the study or investigation. Imaging at early time points, such as the status after a few days of therapy, helps to identify patients with poor response and adverse prognosis which could not be identified using traditional response parameters.

Scans at later time points, such as pre-maintenance or at the time point of achieving CR or MRD-negativity could identify patients with residual disease at locations that were not reached by biopsy, who may benefit from prolonged or intensified treatment. Yet, we need to emphasize that functional imaging data during follow-up is still scarce and the best time point for imaging has yet to be identified.

Sensitivity, Specificity, and Standardization of Imaging for Response Evaluation

Compared to DW-MRI, FDG PET-CT is less sensitive for detection of MM disease at baseline and during follow-up. But what about the sensitivity of functional imaging in general in the context of deep responses to treatment? We recently showed that only 4 of 34 (12%) first-line CR patients who were MRD-negative at a sensitivity level of 1×10^{-5} still presented with FLs in functional imaging. On the other hand, 39/49 (80%) NDMM patients in MRD-positive CR were negative in FDG PET-CT and DW-MRI. Alonso et al. who compared FDG PET-CT to flow cytometry in patients achieving CR showed very similar results, with only 19% of MRD-negative patients being imaging-positive and 82% of MRD-positive patients being FDG PET-negative [48].

Limited sensitivity of functional imaging for detection of residual tumor foci in deep responders is not surprising. For FDG PET-CT, a FL is defined as an area of increased FDG uptake compared to its surroundings or the liver. Thus, tumor cells with a low glucose metabolism (e.g., inactive/dormant cells) would not be detectable. Furthermore, a size-cutoff of 5 mm is usually used to call a FL in functional imaging [17]. Since DW-MRI relies on increased cellularity, a sphere-like tightly packed FL detectable by this method would contain several million cells. Thus, only FLs or EMD mainly consisting of treatment-resistant tumor cells and/or actively growing FLs would be detectable during follow-up, but not a lesion where there are tumor cells that are either dormant or intermingled with other, i.e., hematopoietic or fat cells. Yet, we need to emphasize that this scenario – actively growing FLs in the absence of tumor cells at the iliac crest – occurs in deep-responding NDMM patients and is frequently seen in late-stage patients responding to salvage therapy, making functional imaging an important tool for response evaluation despite limited sensitivity [11].

Specificity is another factor that needs to be considered if functional imaging is to be used for response evaluation. At diagnosis of MM, specificity of FDG PET-CT and DW-MRI in detecting myelomatous involvement has been reported to be ~90% [49–51]. Yet, to the best of our knowledge, specificity for detection of FL in MM patients achieving deep responses has not been reported. There are multiple potential confounders of signals in FDG PET-CT and/or DW-MRI, such as bone marrow hyperplasia due to application of GCSF or recovery of the BM after chemotherapy, inflammation, return of adipocytes in responding BM, metallic implants, and mechanical stress at joints [52]. For DW-MRI, using more sophisticated methods may improve our understanding of ADC value changes during treatment, resulting in more accurate interpretations of DWI images [53]. Furthermore, we showed that the spleen signal on DW-MRI could be useful to discriminate between malignant and nonmalignant/reactive BM hyperintensities [54].

Only recently, there have been initiatives to define standards for monitoring residual disease using functional imaging. Analogous to the Deauville criteria for lymphoma, the IMWG proposed a five-point scoring system for FDG PET-CT [55]. According to these criteria, imaging response is defined as the disappearance of increased FDG uptake found at baseline, or a preceding PET-CT; or a decrease to less than the mediastinal blood pool SUV; or a decrease to less than that of surrounding normal tissue. A score of one or two corresponds to a complete metabolic response. For DW-MRI, guidelines were published by Messiou and co-workers [53]. The authors provide helpful advices regarding data acquisition and analysis and also propose a five-point scoring system for response assessment using the following categories for each anatomical region: (1) highly likely to be responding, (2) likely to be responding, (3) stable, (4) likely to be progressing, and (5) highly likely to be progressing. For more details regarding criteria which define these categories, we refer to this excellent publication. Yet, despite these efforts, we are far from using these methods in clinical routine, since both FDG PET-CT and DW-MRI are poorly available in the clinical setting, reimbursement by health insurances is a critical issue, confirmatory literature is limited, and there have been only a few studies that compared the two methods, among others. In general, due to limited sensitivity and the high number of potential confounders, we would like to emphasize that extensive experience in FDG PET-CT and/or DW-MRI is a prerequisite for response evaluation using functional imaging. The IMWG states that response assessments should be conservative and expects that prospectively collected imaging data will lead to better cutoffs for defining absence of disease on functional imaging scans [17].

Together, limited sensitivity and specificity need to be considered if functional imaging is to be used for response evaluation. Several guidelines for monitoring of residual disease have recently been published, but functional imaging is not a standardized approach yet.

Clinical Consequences

The question arises whether functional imaging results can already be used to guide treatment decisions, e.g., if we would treat a patient with residual active focal lesions differently. Except for progressive disease, the IMWG does not recommend change of treatment solely based on follow-up imaging results, since imaging cannot replace biopsies [17]. Residual FLs on FDG PET-CT or DW-MRI can reflect suboptimal disease control, but we agree with the IMWG that the presence of these lesions alone should not result in change of treatment outside of clinical trials. Occurrence of lesions which are highly suspicious for EMD is an exception, because EMD frequently progresses without systemic or serological progression and is often difficult to reach by biopsy [13, 56, 57]. Thus, new EMD lesions could well trigger initiation of new therapies. We also think that patients with newly occurring intramedullary FDG-avid FLs during treatment should at least be considered for treatment intensification, especially high-risk patients. Here, new lesions herald dismal outcome and rapid relapse (own unpublished observations). Furthermore, we have shown that patients in CR, who are MRD-AND imaging-positive, have such a dismal outcome that switching to alternative treatments could be beneficial [11]. We are fully aware that false-positive results in functional imaging do occur frequently and that a subsequent scan will be required to confirm new FLs. We also appreciate that prospective trials are required to support the idea of treatment intensification or change based on imaging scans. Yet, in the world of clinical trials where MRD diagnostics results are increasingly being used as surrogate markers for outcome, we strongly believe in imaging as a complementary strategy to adjust for spatial differences in response and we recommend not relying on data from a single BM site.

Conclusions

In theory, functional imaging allows for a noninvasive monitoring of treatment activity and response and may help overcome the limitations of conventional response evaluation in patients with non-secretory or extramedullary disease. Indeed, these techniques account for the heterogenous disease distribution in MM patient and complement single-sited MRD diagnostics based on highly sensitive approaches. However, functional imaging is not a standardized approach yet, and accuracy is a variable that needs to be considered, especially in deep responders. Recent guidelines for response evaluation using functional imaging are an important first step, but larger prospective studies and international efforts are required, with the aim to standardize acquisition and interpretation of scans, if these techniques are to be integrated in clinical trials as well as in daily clinical practice.

Competing Interests The authors declare no conflict of interest.

Funding This work was funded by the BMBF (FKZ 01KD1906). LR was funded by the Deutsche Krebshilfe via the MSNZ program Würzburg and the Interdisciplinary Center for Clinical Research Würzburg (IZKF). NW was supported by the Dietmar-Hopp-Stiftung GmbH (1DH118373, Universitätsklinikum Heidelberg und 1DH1911364, DKFZ).

References

1. Dutoit JC, Vanderkerken MA, Verstraete KL. Value of whole body MRI and dynamic contrast enhanced MRI in the diagnosis, follow-up and evaluation of disease activity and extent in multiple myeloma. Eur J Radiol. 2013;82(9):1444–52.
2. Walker R, Barlogie B, Haessler J, Tricot G, Anaissie E, Shaughnessy JD Jr, et al. Magnetic resonance imaging in multiple myeloma: diagnostic and clinical implications. J Clin Oncol. 2007;25(9):1121–8.
3. Rasche L, Buros A, Weinhold N, Stein CK, McDonald JE, Chavan SS, et al. The clinical impact of macrofocal disease in multiple myeloma differs between presentation and relapse. Blood. 2016;128(22):4431.
4. Dimopoulos MA, Pouli A, Anagnostopoulos A, Repoussis P, Symeonidis A, Terpos E, et al. Macrofocal multiple myeloma in young patients: a distinct entity with favorable prognosis. Leuk Lymphoma. 2006;47(8):1553–6.
5. Dores GM, Landgren O, McGlynn KA, Curtis RE, Linet MS, Devesa SS. Plasmacytoma of bone, extramedullary plasmacytoma, and multiple myeloma: incidence and survival in the United States, 1992–2004. Br J Haematol. 2009;144(1):86–94.
6. Zamagni E, Patriarca F, Nanni C, Zannetti B, Englaro E, Pezzi A, et al. Prognostic relevance of 18-F FDG PET/CT in newly diagnosed multiple myeloma patients treated with up-front autologous transplantation. Blood. 2011;118(23):5989–95.
7. Waheed S, Mitchell A, Usmani S, Epstein J, Yaccoby S, Nair B, et al. Standard and novel imaging methods for multiple myeloma:

correlates with prognostic laboratory variables including gene expression profiling data. Haematologica. 2013;98(1):71–8.
8. Matsue K, Kobayashi H, Matsue Y, Abe Y, Narita K, Kitadate A, et al. Prognostic significance of bone marrow abnormalities in the appendicular skeleton of patients with multiple myeloma. Blood Adv. 2018;2(9):1032–9.
9. Rasche L, Angtuaco E, McDonald JE, Buros A, Stein C, Pawlyn C, et al. Low expression of hexokinase-2 is associated with false-negative FDG-positron emission tomography in multiple myeloma. Blood. 2017;130(1):30–4.
10. Rasche L, Angtuaco EJ, Alpe TL, Gershner GH, McDonald JE, Samant RS, et al. The presence of large focal lesions is a strong independent prognostic factor in multiple myeloma. Blood. 2018;132(1):59–66.
11. Rasche L, Alapat D, Kumar M, Gershner G, McDonald J, Wardell CP, et al. Combination of flow cytometry and functional imaging for monitoring of residual disease in myeloma. Leukemia. 2019;33:1713.
12. Rasche L, Kortum KM, Raab MS, Weinhold N. The impact of tumor heterogeneity on diagnostics and novel therapeutic strategies in multiple myeloma. Int J Mol Sci. 2019;20(5):1248.
13. Rasche L, Bernard C, Topp MS, Kapp M, Duell J, Wesemeier C, et al. Features of extramedullary myeloma relapse: high proliferation, minimal marrow involvement, adverse cytogenetics: a retrospective single-center study of 24 cases. Ann Hematol. 2012;91(7):1031–7.
14. Rasche L, Rollig C, Stuhler G, Danhof S, Mielke S, Grigoleit GU, et al. Allogeneic hematopoietic cell transplantation in multiple myeloma: focus on longitudinal assessment of donor chimerism, extramedullary disease, and high-risk cytogenetic features. Biol Blood Marrow Transplant. 2016;22(11):1988–96.
15. Durie BG, Harousseau JL, Miguel JS, Blade J, Barlogie B, Anderson K, et al. International uniform response criteria for multiple myeloma. Leukemia. 2006;20(9):1467–73.
16. Kumar S, Paiva B, Anderson KC, Durie B, Landgren O, Moreau P, et al. International Myeloma Working Group consensus criteria for response and minimal residual disease assessment in multiple myeloma. Lancet Oncol. 2016;17(8):e328–46.
17. Hillengass J, Usmani S, Rajkumar SV, Durie BGM, Mateos MV, Lonial S, et al. International myeloma working group consensus recommendations on imaging in monoclonal plasma cell disorders. Lancet Oncol. 2019;20(6):e302–e12.

18. Bauerle T, Hillengass J, Fechtner K, Zechmann CM, Grenacher L, Moehler TM, et al. Multiple myeloma and monoclonal gammopathy of undetermined significance: importance of whole-body versus spinal MR imaging. Radiology. 2009;252(2):477–85.
19. Seaman ME, Contino G, Bardeesy N, Kelly KA. Molecular imaging agents: impact on diagnosis and therapeutics in oncology. Expert Rev Mol Med. 2010;12:e20.
20. Barwick T, Bretsztajn L, Wallitt K, Amiras D, Rockall A, Messiou C. Imaging in myeloma with focus on advanced imaging techniques. Br J Radiol. 2019;92(1095):20180768.
21. Moulopoulos LA, Koutoulidis V, Hillengass J, Zamagni E, Aquerreta JD, Roche CL, et al. Recommendations for acquisition, interpretation and reporting of whole body low dose CT in patients with multiple myeloma and other plasma cell disorders: a report of the IMWG Bone Working Group. Blood Cancer J. 2018;8(10):95.
22. Moreau P, Attal M, Caillot D, Macro M, Karlin L, Garderet L, et al. Prospective evaluation of magnetic resonance imaging and [(18)F]Fluorodeoxyglucose positron emission tomography-computed tomography at diagnosis and before maintenance therapy in symptomatic patients with multiple myeloma included in the IFM/DFCI 2009 trial: results of the IMAJEM study. J Clin Oncol. 2017;35(25):2911–8.
23. Hillengass J, Ayyaz S, Kilk K, Weber MA, Hielscher T, Shah R, et al. Changes in magnetic resonance imaging before and after autologous stem cell transplantation correlate with response and survival in multiple myeloma. Haematologica. 2012;97(11):1757–60.
24. Merz M, Hielscher T, Mai EK, Seckinger A, Hose D, Jauch A, et al. Cystic transformation of focal lesions after therapy is associated with remission but adverse outcome in myeloma. Blood Cancer J. 2019;9(9):71.
25. Bartel TB, Haessler J, Brown TL, Shaughnessy JD Jr, van Rhee F, Anaissie E, et al. F18-fluorodeoxyglucose positron emission tomography in the context of other imaging techniques and prognostic factors in multiple myeloma. Blood. 2009;114(10):2068–76.
26. Zamagni E, Nanni C, Mancuso K, Tacchetti P, Pezzi A, Pantani L, et al. PET/CT improves the definition of complete response and allows to detect otherwise unidentifiable skeletal progression in multiple myeloma. Clin Cancer Res. 2015;21(19):4384–90.

27. Ripani D, Caldarella C, Za T, Pizzuto DA, Rossi E, De Stefano V, et al. Prognostic significance of normalized FDG-PET parameters in patients with multiple myeloma undergoing induction chemotherapy and autologous hematopoietic stem cell transplantation: a retrospective single-center evaluation. Eur J Nucl Med Mol Imaging. 2019;46(1):116–28.
28. Sundaram S, Driscoll J, Fernandez-Ulloa M, de Lima M, Malek E. FDG PET imaging in multiple myeloma: implications for response assessments in clinical trials. Am J Nucl Med Mol Imaging. 2018;8(6):421–7.
29. Nanni C, Zamagni E, Celli M, Caroli P, Ambrosini V, Tacchetti P, et al. The value of 18F-FDG PET/CT after autologous stem cell transplantation (ASCT) in patients affected by multiple myeloma (MM): experience with 77 patients. Clin Nucl Med. 2013;38(2):e74–9.
30. Stolzenburg A, Luckerath K, Samnick S, Speer M, Kneer K, Schmid JS, et al. Prognostic value of [(18)F]FDG-PET/CT in multiple myeloma patients before and after allogeneic hematopoietic cell transplantation. Eur J Nucl Med Mol Imaging. 2018;45(10):1694–704.
31. Lapa C, Luckerath K, Malzahn U, Samnick S, Einsele H, Buck AK, et al. 18 FDG-PET/CT for prognostic stratification of patients with multiple myeloma relapse after stem cell transplantation. Oncotarget. 2014;5(17):7381–91.
32. Kwee TC, Takahara T, Ochiai R, Nievelstein RA, Luijten PR. Diffusion-weighted whole-body imaging with background body signal suppression (DWIBS): features and potential applications in oncology. Eur Radiol. 2008;18(9):1937–52.
33. Giles SL, Messiou C, Collins DJ, Morgan VA, Simpkin CJ, West S, et al. Whole-body diffusion-weighted MR imaging for assessment of treatment response in myeloma. Radiology. 2014;271(3):785–94.
34. Horger M, Weisel K, Horger W, Mroue A, Fenchel M, Lichy M. Whole-body diffusion-weighted MRI with apparent diffusion coefficient mapping for early response monitoring in multiple myeloma: preliminary results. AJR Am J Roentgenol. 2011;196(6):W790–5.
35. Fenchel M, Konaktchieva M, Weisel K, Kraus S, Claussen CD, Horger M. Response assessment in patients with multiple myeloma during antiangiogenic therapy using arterial spin labeling and diffusion-weighted imaging: a feasibility study. Acad Radiol. 2010;17(11):1326–33.

36. Messiou C, Giles S, Collins DJ, West S, Davies FE, Morgan GJ, et al. Assessing response of myeloma bone disease with diffusion-weighted MRI. Br J Radiol. 2012;85(1020):e1198–203.
37. Abe Y, Ikeda S, Kitadate A, Narita K, Kobayashi H, Miura D, et al. Low hexokinase-2 expression-associated false-negative (18)F-FDG PET/CT as a potential prognostic predictor in patients with multiple myeloma. Eur J Nucl Med Mol Imaging. 2019;46(6):1345–50.
38. Lapa C, Schreder M, Schirbel A, Samnick S, Kortum KM, Herrmann K, et al. [68Ga]Pentixafor-PET/CT for imaging of chemokine receptor CXCR4 expression in multiple myeloma – comparison to [18F]FDG and laboratory values. Theranostics. 2017;7(1):205–12.
39. Lapa C, Knop S, Schreder M, Rudelius M, Knott M, Jorg G, et al. 11C-methionine-PET in multiple myeloma: correlation with clinical parameters and bone marrow involvement. Theranostics. 2016;6(2):254–61.
40. Lapa C, Kircher M, Da Via M, Schreder M, Rasche L, Kortum KM, et al. Comparison of 11C-choline and 11C-methionine PET/CT in multiple myeloma. Clin Nucl Med. 2019;44(8):620–4.
41. Jamet B, Bailly C, Carlier T, Touzeau C, Nanni C, Zamagni E, et al. Interest of pet imaging in multiple myeloma. Front Med (Lausanne). 2019;6:69.
42. Sachpekidis C, Goldschmidt H, Hose D, Pan L, Cheng C, Kopka K, et al. PET/CT studies of multiple myeloma using (18) F-FDG and (18) F-NaF: comparison of distribution patterns and tracers' pharmacokinetics. Eur J Nucl Med Mol Imaging. 2014;41(7):1343–53.
43. Caserta E, Chea J, Minnix M, Poku EK, Viola D, Vonderfecht S, et al. Copper 64-labeled daratumumab as a PET/CT imaging tracer for multiple myeloma. Blood. 2018;131(7):741–5.
44. Usmani SZ, Mitchell A, Waheed S, Crowley J, Hoering A, Petty N, et al. Prognostic implications of serial 18-fluoro-deoxyglucose emission tomography in multiple myeloma treated with total therapy 3. Blood. 2013;121(10):1819–23.
45. Bailly C, Carlier T, Jamet B, Eugene T, Touzeau C, Attal M, et al. Interim PET analysis in first-line therapy of multiple myeloma: prognostic value of DeltaSUVmax in the FDG-avid patients of the IMAJEM study. Clin Cancer Res. 2018;24(21):5219–24.
46. Mosebach J, Shah S, Delorme S, Hielscher T, Goldschmidt H, Schlemmer HP, et al. Prognostic significance of tumor burden assessed by whole-body magnetic resonance imaging in multiple

myeloma patients treated with allogeneic stem cell transplantation. Haematologica. 2018;103(2):336–43.
47. Davies FE, Rosenthal A, Rasche L, Petty NM, McDonald JE, Ntambi JA, et al. Treatment to suppression of focal lesions on positron emission tomography-computed tomography is a therapeutic goal in newly diagnosed multiple myeloma. Haematologica. 2018;103(6):1047–53.
48. Alonso R, Cedena MT, Gomez-Grande A, Rios R, Moraleda JM, Cabanas V, et al. Imaging and bone marrow assessments improve minimal residual disease prediction in multiple myeloma. Am J Hematol. 2019;94(8):853–61.
49. Bredella MA, Steinbach L, Caputo G, Segall G, Hawkins R. Value of FDG PET in the assessment of patients with multiple myeloma. AJR Am J Roentgenol. 2005;184(4):1199–204.
50. Hillengass J, Bauerle T, Bartl R, Andrulis M, McClanahan F, Laun FB, et al. Diffusion-weighted imaging for non-invasive and quantitative monitoring of bone marrow infiltration in patients with monoclonal plasma cell disease: a comparative study with histology. Br J Haematol. 2011;153(6):721–8.
51. Messiou C, Collins DJ, Morgan VA, Desouza NM. Optimising diffusion weighted MRI for imaging metastatic and myeloma bone disease and assessing reproducibility. Eur Radiol. 2011;21(8):1713–8.
52. Lin WC, Chen JH. Pitfalls and limitations of diffusion-weighted magnetic resonance imaging in the diagnosis of urinary bladder cancer. Transl Oncol. 2015;8(3):217–30.
53. Messiou C, Hillengass J, Delorme S, Lecouvet FE, Moulopoulos LA, Collins DJ, et al. Guidelines for acquisition, interpretation, and reporting of whole-body MRI in myeloma: myeloma response assessment and diagnosis system (MY-RADS). Radiology. 2019;291(1):5–13.
54. Rasche L, Kumar M, Gershner G, Samant R, Van Hemert R, Heidemeier A, et al. Lack of spleen signal on diffusion weighted MRI is associated with high tumor burden and poor prognosis in multiple myeloma: a link to extramedullary hematopoiesis? Theranostics. 2019;9(16):4756–63.
55. Nanni C, Versari A, Chauvie S, Bertone E, Bianchi A, Rensi M, et al. Interpretation criteria for FDG PET/CT in multiple myeloma (IMPeTUs): final results. IMPeTUs (Italian myeloma criteria for PET USe). Eur J Nucl Med Mol Imaging. 2018;45(5):712–9.

56. Kumar AK, Dakhil C, Teeka Satyan M, Haideri N. Extramedullary progression of multiple myeloma despite concomitant medullary response to multiple combination therapies and autologous transplant: a case report. J Med Case Rep. 2014;8:299.
57. Terpos E, Rezvani K, Basu S, Milne AE, Rose PE, Scott GL, et al. Plasmacytoma relapses in the absence of systemic progression post-high-dose therapy for multiple myeloma. Eur J Haematol. 2005;75(5):376–83.

Chapter 6
New Perspectives in Imaging Techniques

Bastien Jamet, Clément Bailly, Thomas Carlier, Anne-Victoire Michaud, Cyrille Touzeau, Philippe Moreau, Caroline Bodet-Milin, and Françoise Kraeber-Bodéré

B. Jamet (✉) · A.-V. Michaud
Nuclear Medicine Unit, University Hospital, Nantes, France
e-mail: bastien.jamet@chu-nantes.fr;
anne-victoire.michaud@chu-nantes.fr

C. Bailly · T. Carlier · C. Bodet-Milin
Nuclear Medicine Unit, University Hospital, Nantes, France

CRCINA, INSERM, CNRS, Angers University, Nantes University, Nantes, France
e-mail: clement.bailly@chu-nantes.fr; thomas.carlier@chu-nantes.fr;
caroline.milin@chu-nantes.fr

C. Touzeau · P. Moreau
CRCINA, INSERM, CNRS, Angers University, Nantes University, Nantes, France

Haematology Department, University Hospital, Nantes, France
e-mail: cyrille.touzeau@chu-nantes.fr; philippe.moreau@chu-nantes.fr

F. Kraeber-Bodéré
Nuclear Medicine Unit, University Hospital, Nantes, France

CRCINA, INSERM, CNRS, Angers University, Nantes University, Nantes, France

Nuclear Medicine Unit, ICO-Gauducheau, Nantes-Saint-Herblain, France
e-mail: francoise.bodere@chu-nantes.fr

E. Zamagni (ed.), *Management of Bone Disease and Kidney Failure in Multiple Myeloma*,
https://doi.org/10.1007/978-3-030-63662-3_6

Modern imaging including whole-body computed tomography (WBCT), 18F-fluorodeoxyglucose (FDG)-positron emission tomography/computed tomography (FDG-PET/CT), and whole-body magnetic resonance imaging (WBMRI) is now mandatory at multiple myeloma (MM) diagnosis to detect bone (and/or extra-medullary) disease leading to the recommendation to treat these patients. Moreover, FDG-PET/CT is the reference imaging technique for the assessment of response to therapy. However, FDG-PET/CT is negative for 10 to 20% of patients with an initial diagnosis of symptomatic MM [1–2]. Therefore, FDG-PET/CT is not an appropriate tool to evaluate minimal residual disease (MRD) in these MM patients with tumor disease presenting a low avidity for glucose. Other PET tracers and new high sensitive functional MRI approaches are needed for disease detection at baseline and MRD evaluation after therapy.

New PET/CT Tracers

Introduction

FDG is a nontumor-specific metabolic tracer. Indeed, inflammatory cells are also avid for glucose and are therefore likely to generate false-positive images. Moreover, tumors' avidity for glucose and therefore for FDG is variable: aggressive, fast-growing lesions are avid for glucose and therefore well visualized, but indolent or dormant cells, often observed in bone niches in MM, consuming less glucose may be more difficult to detect. In that respect, a study of 227 patients with the initial diagnosis of symptomatic MM reported an 11% FDG-PET/CT negativity rate [1]. In this subgroup, a low expression of the hexokinase 2 gene (which catalyzes the first stage of glycolysis) was noted. Abe et al. recently confirmed this observation with 12% negative FDG-PET/CT associated with low expression of hexokinase 2 and reported better prognosis in these patients [2]. In this context, the development of new PET imaging tracers, more sensitive and specific than FDG, appears essential to improve detection of MRD by targeting other metabolic pathways or biomarkers expressed by neoplasm's cells.

Exploration of Metabolic Pathways

The use of 11C-methionine (MET), an amino-acid PET tracer whose uptake reflects the increased protein synthesis of malignant cells, has been reported. Studies performed by Lapa et al. and Okasaki et al., assessing MET, showed a good correlation with bone marrow infiltration and a higher sensitivity than FDG to detect intra- and extramedullary MM lesions at baseline or at relapse [3, 4]. Nevertheless, the prognostic value of this tracer is questionable, especially in comparison with FDG.

Choline is a lipid PET tracer clinically used for the evaluation of relapse of prostate cancer. Cassou et al. have compared the respective sensitivities of FDG and 18fluorocholine (FCH) for the detection of focal lesions at disease relapse or progression, in a small series of patients [5]. In this study, 76% more lesions were detected with FCH, suggesting the superior diagnostic potential of this tracer for MM relapse/progression exploration. However, in this small cohort, no strictly FDG PET/CT-negative and FCH PET-positive cases were reported. Moreover, unfavorable physiological biodistribution (increased background of the liver parenchyma and of the bone marrow) could appear as a limitation.

The performance of another lipid tracer, 11C-Acetate, was reported in a preliminary study at diagnosis in symptomatic MM patients [6]. This study showed that 11C-acetate performed significantly better than FDG in the detection of both diffuse and focal MM with higher uptake. This result is promising, but needs to be verified in a larger number of patients, including relapsing MM patients.

18F-Fludarabine (2-[18F]fluoro-9-β-D-arabinofuranosyl-adenine) represents also a good potential candidate for the exploration of MM. Indeed, based on work already published in lymphoma models, this tracer has a high selectivity for lymphoid cells, independently of the cell cycle [7–10]. Preclinical studies performed in mice comparing the distribution of 18F-fludarabine and FDG showed a significantly lower uptake of 18-fludarabine in inflammatory cells, a very rapid emptying in the physiological uptake sites of FDG, and finally a better correlation between uptake and histology than FDG. The results of a first pilot clinical study carried out in 10 patients newly diagnosed with lymphomas (diffuse large cell B lymphomas and chronic lymphoid leukemia) confirmed all the results obtained in preclinical studies as well as the excellent clinical tolerability of the tracer [10]. Indeed, this pilot study demonstrated the good sensitivity of 18F-Fludarabine to detect lymphomatous lesions, particularly in indolent lymphomas. It confirmed the absence of uptake on inflammatory lesions and thus the probable interest in terms of specificity, particularly for the evaluation of the therapeutic response. Given these relevant results in lymphopathies, the feasibility of using 18F-Fludarabine in a pre-clinical model of MM was performed, in comparison with FDG [11]. The results of this work confirmed the good uptake of 18F-fludarabine in the 5 xenograft mice explored in imaging. A better correlation between the tumor volume evaluated with bioluminescence and the uptake of the radiopharmaceutical was found with 18F-fludarabine than with FDG. Finally, the results of immunohistochemical analyses evaluating CD138 and F4/80 expression (to characterize inflammatory cells) suggested a better specificity of 18F-fludarabine than FDG for MM.

Conversely, despite its potential theoretical value, discouraging results were observed regarding the performance of 18F-NaF in the evaluation of MM [12, 13]. This radiotracer, which reflects bone remodeling, appears to be an interesting imaging method for malignant bone diseases. However, as reported in diagnostic and treatment evaluation, 18F-NaF does not appear to add significant information to FDG-PET in MM patients.

Similar discouraging results were described with hypoxia tracers in MM, despite interesting data in solid tumors, such as head and neck cancers and non-small cell lung cancers. The PET tracer 1-α-D: –(5-deoxy-5-[18F]-fluoroarabinofuranosyl)-2-nitroimidazole (18F-FAZA) was evaluated in five patients diagnosed with relapsing MM based on a positive FDG-PET [14]. No significant uptake of [18 F]-FAZA was observed in any of the patients, despite the presence of focal disease. These findings might suggest that the degree of hypoxia is not substantially different in MM lesions compared to the surrounding bone marrow compartment.

Phenotype Tumor Imaging

Benefiting of major technological advances, molecular characterization of tumors has helped highlight biomarkers, useful in identifying cancer cells and understanding the variability of response to therapeutic agents. Moreover, these biomarkers can also be used as targets and have thus enabled the development of more specific targeted therapies. In medical practice, the identification of these biomarkers slowly but surely becomes a prerequisite before any treatment decision, leading to the concept of precision medicine. The development of phenotype tumor PET imaging with monoclonal antibodies (mAbs) or peptides thus offers a noninvasive solution to assess in vivo target expression and distribution and to obtain reliable diagnostic, prognostic, and theranostic information. Consistent preclinical and clinical studies have been performed showing the potential for proper estimation of the probe biodistribution of immuno-PET before radioimmunotherapy (RIT) [15]. Indeed, by translating tumor-to-background ratios into potential absorbed radiation doses, this approach allows for improved optimal dosing for personalized medicine in the context of multimodality treatment strategies.

In MM, among the interesting targets, cluster of differentiation 38 (CD38) and CD138 is highly expressed on myeloma cells, but at relatively low levels on normal hematopoietic cells. These glycoproteins functioning in cell adhesion and signal transduction are currently used as standard markers in many laboratories for the identification and purification of myeloma cells. Anti-CD38 or anti-CD138 immuno-PET thus has the potential to improve MM imaging, especially regarding lesions with low metabolic activity. In preclinical studies, mAbs targeting these two biomarkers labeled with zirconium 89 or 64 copper showed excellent results with efficient binding and high uptake in MM lesions [16–19]. These findings have been corroborated by Ulaner et al. in a first-in-human phase I trial where excellent targeting of MM was observed [20]. The evaluation of this imaging related to response to treatment and MRD assessment will be particularly interesting. Moreover, these immuno-PET imaging could also be considered as a companion agent for currently developed targeted therapies (precision therapeutics probes). An anti-CD38 human monoclonal antibody, daratumab, has indeed been developed with promising results and a recent FDA approval [21]. Phase I–II studies have been also initiated with an anti-CD138 mAb [22, 23]. Furthermore, as previously demonstrated with radiolabeled anti-CD20 mAb in lymphoma [24], stronger response might be obtained in the context of RIT. Preclinical studies have already been performed in mice models with alpha emitting 213 bismuth (213 Bi) or 225 actinium (225Ac) radio-immunoconjugates, showing promising results [25–27].

Another new and potentially interesting tracer is CXC chemokine receptor 4 (CXCR4). This protein is implicated in the process of cell migration as well as in the homing process of hematopoietic stem cells to the bone marrow compartment. It is expressed in high density by approximately 50% of the MM monoclonal plasma cells and is associated to disease progression and poor prognosis. A recent study has revealed the potential of 68Ga-Pentixafor, a labelled peptide with high affinity for CXCR4 and an excellent signal-to-noise ratio in CXCR4-expressing patients [28]. This same ligand can also be labelled with therapeutic ß-emitters such as 177Lutetium or

90Yttrium, with good tolerance of the treatment and very encouraging high initial response rates in advanced MM cases [29].

New Functional MRI

Diffusion-Weighted MRI

Introduction

Diffusion-weighted magnetic resonance imaging (DW-MRI) produces images reflecting differences of motion of water at a cellular level in tissues. Water motion in tissues can occur in intracellular, transmembrane, extracellular, and intravascular compartments. The choice of diffusion weighting (b value) influences the sensitivity to water diffusion in the different compartments. Low b values are sensitive to large diffusion distances, such as flow in blood vessels. Large b values are sensitive to small diffusion distances as extracellular space distances and therefore directly related to cell density. Theoretically, with very large b values (> 4000 s/mm^2), it is possible to illustrate the movement of intracellular water protons, but this is extremely challenging. Imaging with more than one b value allows automated calculation of the apparent diffusion coefficient (ADC) for each voxel in the image, and a quantitative map can be produced. Tumor (tightly packed cells) therefore appears as area of restriction of water diffusion (high signal on source diffusion image and low value on ADC map). Response to therapy induces decrease of cellularity so diminishing signal at high b value and increase of ADC values. In MM, it has been shown that b values of around 1400 smm^{-2} are optimal for maximizing contrast between normal and infiltrated bone [30]. However, technical challenges to achieve such high b values are resulting b value of 900 smm^{-2} are often chosen as a compromise between robust data and whole-body (WB) coverage achievable in a reasonable time frame. The excellent image contrast between normal and diseased bone marrow by DW-MRI leads to superior lesion detection compared to conventional morphological (included STIR) and contrast-enhanced MRI sequences [31–33].

DW-MRI for Disease Detection Vs FDG-PET/CT

DW-MRI seems to be a highly sensitive new tool for disease detection in MM. There is no large prospective comparison published yet between WB DW-MRI and WB FDG-PET/CT for detection of intra- and extramedullary disease in MM, especially at initial workup.

A recent retrospective study concerning 49 patients with MM at baseline and at relapse [34] showed WB DW-MRI is more sensitive than FDG-PET/CT for detecting bone lesions, in all regions except the skull, both in patients with a new diagnosis and previously treated, and especially in patients with a low percentage of plasma cells in bone marrow. For detecting extramedullary disease (EMD), WB DW-MRI and FDG-PET/CT had equivalent sensitivity.

In smaller cohorts, Sachpekidis et al. [35] showed in a study of 24 MM patients (15 newly diagnosed, 9 pretreated) WB DW-MRI was more sensitive than FDG-PET/CT for detecting myeloma lesions in the whole population. However, analysis including only the 15 untreated MM patients revealed an equivalent sensitivity of 90% for both FDG-PET/CT and WB DW-MRI and an overall concordance of 72%. Moreover, in a retrospective monocentric study of 17 patients (Pawlyn et al.) [36], WB DW-MRI significantly depicted more bone lesions than FDG-PET/CT in all regions except for pelvis and long bones. Diffuse bone marrow involvement (BMI) was reported in 37% of regions imaged on WB DW-MRI compared with only 7% on FDG-PET/CT.

Performance of DW-MRI for monitoring of residual disease after therapy has been investigated recently by the Little Rock team [37]. In a cohort of 168 patients, flow cytometry, FDG-PET/CT, and DW- MRI were performed at the onset of complete remission (CR) during first-line or salvage therapy.

Compared to PET, DW-MRI detected more patients with residual lesions (21% vs. 6%). Specifically, only six of the DW-MRI-positive patients also presented with focal bone lesions (FLs) in PET. Yet, there were five patients with FLs in PET only, suggesting that the two techniques are complementary. Residual FLs, detectable in 24% of first-line patients, were associated with short PFS. Progression-free survival (PFS) of patients with FLs only detectable using DW-MRI was not significantly different from patients with PET-positive FLs. Combining MRD and imaging improved prediction of outcome, with double-negative and double-positive features defining groups with excellent and dismal PFS, respectively.

DW-MRI for Assessment of Response to Therapy

DW-MRI-derived quantitative biomarker (ADC) has shown interesting results in the attempt of better monitoring response to therapy by MRI.

In a study of Latifoltojar et al. [38], 21 MM patients underwent WB-MRI at diagnosis and after two cycles of chemotherapy. Different quantitative biomarkers were extracted. Of 254 FLs analyzed, signal fat fraction (sFF) and ADC significantly increased in responders but not in nonresponders. However, FL sFF was the best discriminator of treatment response (AUC 1.0), and bone sFF repeatability was excellent (ICC 0.98), better than bone ADC repeatability (ICC 0.47 means more variation in per patient analysis). Indeed, the temporal changes of ADC following myelomatous infiltration and treatment are complex and affected by several factors such as the amount of fatty (yellow) marrow, cell size, bulk flow in capillaries, and cellular architecture [39].

Previously, in a smaller cohort of 12 MM patients, ADC evaluation of FLs and EMD 3 weeks after onset of therapy showed an increase of 63.9% (range, 8.7–211.3%) in all responder ($N = 11$) patients and a decrease of 7.8% in the sole nonresponding patient [40].

Another work of Giles SL et al. [41] about a group of 26 MM patients who underwent pre- and posttreatment DW-MRI imaging showed mean ADC increased in all but 1 of 20 patients who responded to treatment (mean group increase, 19.8%), while ADC decreased in all 5 patients who did not respond to treatment (mean decrease, 3.2%). ADC measurement was repeatable: mean coefficient of variation was 3.8% in a healthy cohort of volunteers and 2.8% in MM patients.

Wu et al. [42], in a Chinese cohort of 17 newly diagnosed MM patients who underwent WB DW-MRI before and after induction chemotherapy (week 20), found ADC percent changes were significantly higher in deep responders (complete response or very good partial response, mean increase of 36.79%) than in non-deep responders (partial response, minimal response, stable disease or progressive disease, mean increase of 11.50%) in per lesion analysis.

Finally, ADC changes after therapy are included in recent MY-RADS MRI guidelines [43] to help define response assessment category. Patients "highly likely to be responding" category includes previously evident lesion showing increase of ADC from <1400 μm^2/sec to >1400 μm^2/sec and > 40% increase in ADC from baseline with corresponding decrease in normalized high *b*-value signal intensity morphologic findings consistent with stable or responding disease. Patients "likely to be responding" category includes previously evident lesions showing increase of ADC from <1000 μm^2/sec to <1400 μm^2/sec and > 25% but <40% increase in ADC from baseline. However, ADC cutoff values should be considered with caution because ADC values are influenced by a lot of parameters, including the choice of *b* values, the diffusion time achievable with diffusion sequences, patient-related cause (susceptibility effects, motion), and technique-related cause (magnetic field strength, coils).

Dynamic Contrast-Enhanced MRI

Introduction

Dynamic contrast-enhanced MRI (DCE-MRI) is a kinetic analysis of the accumulation and distribution of contrast medium (Gadolinium-DTPA) in vivo in the area of interest (in T1-weighted sequence covering the lumbar spine) after a constant pump controlled bolus injection [44]. Information of pharmacokinetic analysis is contained in two parameters: the amplitude A (associated with blood volume) and exchange rate constant k_{ep} (surrogate for vessel permeability and perfusion), calculated within manually drawn regions of interest.

Bone marrow angiogenesis plays a crucial role in the pathogenesis of MM, is linked to MM-related bone disease, and has a pejorative prognostic significance [45–47]. DCE-MRI helps to study bone marrow microcirculation in patients with MM and asymptomatic precursor diseases [48, 49].

Prognostic Value of DCE-MRI

In a prospective study of Merz et al. [50], DCE-MRI of the lumbar spine was performed in 131 patients with symptomatic newly diagnosed MM. Amplitude A and k_{ep} were positively associated with beta2-microglobulin. Additionally, amplitude A was negatively correlated with hemoglobin levels, and k_{ep} was positively correlated with LDH levels. Higher baseline k_{ep} values were associated with decreased vertebral height in a second MRI, and A values were associated with new vertebral fractures in the lower lumbar spine. Multivariate analysis revealed that amplitude A is an independent adverse risk factor for overall survival.

In an another study of the same group [51] interesting to DCE-MRI parameters of the lumbar spine in 33 healthy controls and 148 patients with monoclonal gammopathy of undetermined significance (MGUS) or smoldering multiple myeloma (SMM), prognostic significance of median of amplitude A and k_{ep} (by multivariate analysis) for time to progression to MM of 79 patients with SMM was found but not in individuals with MGUS. Patients with amplitude A above the optimal cut-off point of 0.89 arbitrary units had a 2-year progression rate into symptomatic disease of 80%.

Another approach of DCE-MRI is proposed in a retrospective 219 patient's study of Dutoit et al. [52], interesting to MGUS (n = 70), MM active disease (n = 126, including new diagnosis of MM and relapse disease), and MM remission (n = 23). DCE-MRI was performed from the first thoracic vertebra to the sacrum. ROIs were manually placed in the aorta, paravertebral muscle, and third lumbar vertebra (L3) for perfusion analysis. A time-intensity curve (TIC) was then created for the selected spinal bodies which could be compared to the curves of the aorta and muscle. Semi-quantitative parameters were derived from the TIC, reflecting the passage of contrast medium from the intravascular space to the interstitial space. A significant correlation was demonstrated between the amount of plasma cells in the bone marrow and the vascularization based on TIC parameters (slope and amplitude wash-in (WI), slope and amplitude wash-out (WO), time to peak (TTP)) which all could also significantly differentiate different subgroups (MGUS, MM active disease, MM remission, and controls). Finally, there was a significant increase of bone marrow perfusion (reflected by slope wash-in of TIU) if MM affected more than 10 skeletal regions with a poorer prognosis. Terpos et al. [53] confirmed the ability of DCE-MRI wash-in perfusion parameter to differentiate symptomatic MM patients to SMM and MGUS patients. Moreover, they found negative correlation between TTP median values and R-ISS values with a subset of patients with low TTP with shorter time to progression compared to all other patients. Finally, TTP was positively correlated with adverse prognostic feature of angiogenesis angiopoietin-1 (Angp-1)/(Angp-2) ratio (reduced in symptomatic MM compared to SMM and MGUS patients).

DCE-MRI for Assessment of Response to Therapy

In the retrospective study of Dutoit et al. [52] mentioned above, a subgroup analysis on 21 patients with active MM disease was conducted, comparing the DCE-MRI results before and 100 days after transplantation. A decrease in bone marrow plasmocytosis (−89%) and monoclonal protein (−68%) was observed. Accordingly, there was a significant decrease of values of slope and amplitude WI with respectively −75% and – 59% and a significant increase of +30% for TTP.

In a larger study of 91 newly diagnosed MM patients [54], DCE-MRI was performed (according to the two-compartment model to quantify amplitude A and exchange rate constant k_{ep}) before and after primary treatment (high-dose therapy with autologous stem cell transplantation (ASCT)). Nonresponders showed significantly higher A values before the start of therapy compared with responders. Lower values for k_{ep} after treatment were found only in responders. Depth of response was significantly correlated to decreased bone marrow microcirculation. Indeed, patients in near complete response (nCR) or complete response (CR) after treatment showed significantly lower values for A compared with patients not achieving nCR + CR. Moreover, higher k_{ep} values at second MRI were positively correlated to shorter overall survival.

In the study of Latifoltojar et al. [38], among different quantitative biomarkers extracted from WB-MRI, FL enhancement after two cycles of bortezomib-based chemotherapy was the worst discriminator because no significant change following treatment was found in responder group.

Conclusion

In the patients with no or low FDG uptake at initial diagnosis of symptomatic MM, FDG-PET/CT is not an appropriate tool to evaluate MRD. In this population, innovative PET tracers and new high sensitive functional MRI approaches could be relevant. ^{11}C-MET, lipid tracers (such as Choline or acetate), and small molecules such as ^{68}Ga-Pentixafor showed a high diagnostic potential in small cohorts of patients. ^{18}F-fludarabine and phenotype tumor imaging as immuno-PET targeting CD138 and CD38 also showed promising results in preclinical models. New functional MRI approaches as DW- and DCE-MRI are not widespread used in routine yet and are mostly performed in a research setting. However, initial experience with DW-MRI in relatively small numbers of MM patients in different disease phases showed the technique to be highly sensitive, especially in detecting diffuse bone marrow disease. DCE-MRI is also able to provide interesting data at baseline, like predicting vertebral fractures and clinical outcome of MM symptomatic patients or progression to active MM disease in patients with SMM. A significant correlation was also demonstrated between the amount of plasma cells in the bone marrow and the vascularization based on DCE-MRI. Thus simultaneous acquiring of combined additional data provided by different PET tracers and functional MRI approaches with a PET-MRI system will be very useful.

Acknowledgments "This work has been supported in part by grants from the French National Agency for Research called 'Investissements d'Avenir' IRON Labex n° ANR-11-LABX-0018-01 and ArronaxPlus Equipex n° ANR-11-EQPX-0004, and by a grant INCa-DGOS-Inserm_12558 (SIRIC ILIAD)."

Bibliography

1. Rasche L, Angtuaco E, McDonald JE, Buros A, Stein C, Pawlyn C, et al. Low expression of hexokinase-2 is associated with false-negative FDG-positron emission tomography in multiple myeloma. Blood. 2017;130:30–4.
2. Abe Y, Ikeda S, Kitadate A, Narita K, Kobayashi H, Miura D, et al. Low hexokinase-2 expression-associated false-negative 18F-FDG PET/CT as a potential prognostic predictor in patients with multiple myeloma. Eur J Nucl Med Mol Imaging. 2019;46:1345–50.

3. Lapa C, Knop S, Schreder M, Rudelius M, Knott M, Jörg G, et al. 11C-methionine-PET in multiple myeloma: correlation with clinical parameters and bone marrow involvement. Theranostics. 2016;6:254–61.
4. Okasaki M, Kubota K, Minamimoto R, Miyata Y, Morooka M, Ito K, et al. Comparison of (11)C-4′-thiothymidine, (11)C-methionine, and (18)F-FDG PET/CT for the detection of active lesions of multiple myeloma. Ann Nucl Med. 2015;29:224–32.
5. Cassou-Mounat T, Balogova S, Nataf V, Calzada M, Huchet V, Kerrou K, et al. 18F-fluorocholine versus 18F-fluorodeoxyglucose for PET/CT imaging in patients with suspected relapsing or progressive multiple myeloma: a pilot study. Eur J Nucl Med Mol Imaging. 2016;43:1995–2004.
6. Ho C, Chen S, Leung YL, Cheng T, Wong K, Cheung SK, et al. 11C-acetate PET/CT for metabolic characterization of multiple myeloma: a comparative study with 18F-FDG PET/CT. J Nucl Med. 2014;55:749–52.
7. Barré L, Hovhannisyan N, Bodet-Milin C, Kraeber-Bodéré F, Damaj G. [18F]-fludarabine for hematological malignancies. Front Med (Lausanne). 2019;6:77.
8. Hovhannisyan N, Dhilly M, Guillouet S, Leporrier M, Barré L. Comparative analysis between [(18)F]Fludarabine-PET and [(18)F]FDG-PET in a murine model of inflammation. Mol Pharm. 2016;13:2136–9.
9. Hovhannisyan N, Guillouet S, Fillesoye F, Dhilly M, Patin D, Galateau F, et al. Evaluation of the specificity of [(18)F]fludarabine PET/CT in a xenograft model of follicular lymphoma: comparison with [(18)F]FDG and impact of rituximab therapy. EJNMMI Res. 2015;5:23.
10. Chantepie S, Hovhannisyan N, Guillouet S, Pelage J-P, Ibazizene M, Bodet-Milin C, et al. 18F-fludarabine PET for lymphoma imaging: first-in-humans study on DLBCL and CLL patients. J Nucl Med. 2018;59:1380–5.
11. Hovhannisyan N, Dhilly M, Fidalgo M, Fillesoye F, Guillouet S, Sola B, et al. [18F]Fludarabine-PET in a murine model of multiple myeloma. PLoS ONE. 2017;12:e0177125.
12. Sachpekidis C, Goldschmidt H, Hose D, Pan L, Cheng C, Kopka K, et al. PET/CT studies of multiple myeloma using 18 F-FDG and 18 F-NaF: comparison of distribution patterns and tracers' pharmacokinetics. Eur J Nucl Med Mol Imaging. 2014;41:1343–53.

13. Sachpekidis C, Hillengass J, Goldschmidt H, Wagner B, Haberkorn U, Kopka K, et al. Treatment response evaluation with (18)F-FDG PET/CT and (18)F-NaF PET/CT in multiple myeloma patients undergoing high-dose chemotherapy and autologous stem cell transplantation. Eur J Nucl Med Mol Imaging. 2017;44:50–62.
14. De Waal EGM, Slart RHJA, Leene MJ, Kluin PM, Vellenga E. 18F-FDG PET increases visibility of bone lesions in relapsed multiple myeloma: is this hypoxia-driven? Clin Nucl Med. 2015;40:291–6.
15. Bailly C, Cléry P-F, Faivre-Chauvet A, Bourgeois M, Guérard F, Haddad F, et al. Immuno-PET for clinical theranostic approaches. Int J Mol Sci. 2016;18 https://doi.org/10.3390/ijms18010057.
16. Bailly C, Gouard S, Lacombe M, Saëc PR-L, Chalopin B, Bourgeois M, et al. Comparison of immuno-PET of CD138 and PET imaging with 64 CuCl 2 and 18 F-FDG in a preclinical syngeneic model of multiple myeloma. Oncotarget. 2018;5 https://doi.org/10.18632/oncotarget.23886.
17. Bailly C, Gouard S, Guérard F, Chalopin B, Carlier T, Faivre-Chauvet A, et al. What is the best radionuclide for immuno-PET of multiple myeloma? A comparison study between 89Zr- and 64Cu-labeled anti-CD138 in a preclinical syngeneic model. Int J Mol Sci. 2019;20:2564.
18. Ghai A, Maji D, Cho N, Chanswangphuwana C, Rettig M, DiPersio J, et al. Preclinical development of CD38-targeted [89Zr]Zr-DFO-daratumumab for imaging multiple myeloma. J Nucl Med. 2017; https://doi.org/10.2967/jnumed.117.196063.
19. Caserta E, Chea J, Minnix M, Viola D, Vonderfecht S, Yazaki P, et al. Copper-64-labeled daratumumab as a PET/CT imaging tracer for multiple myeloma. Blood. 2018; https://doi.org/10.1182/blood-2017-09-807263.
20. Ulaner G, Sobol N, O'Donoghue J, Burnazi E, Staton K, Weber W, et al. Preclinical development and First-in-human imaging of 89Zr-Daratumumab for CD38 targeted imaging of myeloma. J Nucl Med. 2019;60:203.
21. Plesner T, Krejcik J. Daratumumab for the treatment of multiple myeloma. Front Immunol. 2018;9 https://doi.org/10.3389/fimmu.2018.01228.
22. Heffner LT, Jagannath S, Zimmerman TM, Lee KP, Rosenblatt J, Lonial S, et al. BT062, an antibody-drug conjugate directed against CD138, given weekly for 3 weeks in each 4 week

cycle: safety and further evidence of clinical activity. Blood. 2012;120:4042.
23. Kelly KR, Siegel DS, Chanan-Khan AA, Somlo G, Heffner LT, Jagannath S, et al. Indatuximab ravtansine (BT062) in combination with low-dose dexamethasone and lenalidomide or pomalidomide: clinical activity in patients with relapsed/refractory multiple myeloma. Blood. 2016;128:4486.
24. Rizzieri D. Zevalin(®) (ibritumomab tiuxetan): after more than a decade of treatment experience, what have we learned? Crit Rev Oncol Hematol. 2016;105:5–17.
25. Chérel M, Gouard S, Gaschet J, Saï-Maurel C, Bruchertseifer F, Morgenstern A, et al. 213Bi radioimmunotherapy with an anti-mCD138 monoclonal antibody in a murine model of multiple myeloma. J Nucl Med. 2013;54:1597–604.
26. Fichou N, Gouard S, Maurel C, Barbet J, Ferrer L, Morgenstern A, et al. Single-dose anti-CD138 radioimmunotherapy: bismuth-213 is more efficient than lutetium-177 for treatment of multiple myeloma in a preclinical model. Front Med (Lausanne). 2015;2:76.
27. Green DJ, O'Steen S, Lin Y, Comstock ML, Kenoyer AL, Hamlin DK, et al. CD38 bispecific antibody pretargeted radioimmunotherapy for multiple myeloma and other B cell malignancies. Blood. 2017; https://doi.org/10.1182/blood-2017-09-807,610.
28. Lapa C, Schreder M, Schirbel A, Samnick S, Kortüm KM, Herrmann K, et al. [68Ga]Pentixafor-PET/CT for imaging of chemokine receptor CXCR4 expression in multiple myeloma – comparison to [18F]FDG and laboratory values. Theranostics. 2017;7:205–12.
29. Herrmann K, Schottelius M, Lapa C, Osl T, Poschenrieder A, Hänscheid H, et al. First-in-human experience of CXCR4-directed endoradiotherapy with 177Lu- and 90Y-labeled pentixather in advanced-stage multiple myeloma with extensive intra- and extramedullary disease. J Nucl Med. 2016;57:248–51.
30. Messiou C, Collins DJ, Morgan VA, Desouza NM. Optimising diffusion weighted MRI for imaging metastatic and myeloma bone disease and assessing reproducibility. Eur Radiol. 2011;21(8):1713–8.
31. Pearce T, Philip S, Brown J, Koh DM, Burn PR. Bone metastases from prostate, breast and multiple myeloma: differences in lesion conspicuity at short-tau inversion recovery and diffusion-weighted MRI. Br J Radiol. 2012;85(1016):1102–6.

32. Squillaci E, Bolacchi F, Altobelli S, Franceschini L, Bergamini A, Cantonetti M, et al. Pre-treatment staging of multiple myeloma patients: comparison of whole-body diffusion weighted imaging with whole-body T1-weighted contrast-enhanced imaging. Acta Radiol. 2015;56(6):733–8.
33. Dutoit JC, Vanderkerken MA, Anthonissen J, Dochy F, Verstraete KL. The diagnostic value of SE MRI and DWI of the spine in patients with monoclonal gammopathy of undetermined significance, smouldering myeloma and multiple myeloma. Eur Radiol. 2014;24(11):2754–65.
34. Chen J, Li C, Tian Y, Xiao Q, Deng M, Hu H, et al. Comparison of whole-body DWI and 18F-FDG PET/CT for detecting intramedullary and extramedullary lesions in multiple myeloma. AJR Am J Roentgenol. 2019;213(3):514–23.
35. Sachpekidis C, Mosebach J, Freitag MT, Wilhelm T, Mai EK, Goldschmidt H, et al. Application of (18)F-FDG PET and diffusion weighted imaging (DWI) in multiple myeloma: comparison of functional imaging modalities. Am J Nucl Med Mol Imaging. 2015;5(5):479–92.
36. Pawlyn C, Fowkes L, Otero S, Jones JR, Boyd KD, Davies FE, et al. Whole-body diffusion-weighted MRI: a new gold standard for assessing disease burden in patients with multiple myeloma? Leukemia. 2016;30(6):1446–8.
37. Rasche L, Alapat D, Kumar M, Gershner G, McDonald J, Wardell CP, et al. Combination of flow cytometry and functional imaging for monitoring of residual disease in myeloma. Leukemia. *2019*;33(7):1713–22.
38. Latifoltojar A, Hall-Craggs M, Bainbridge A, Rabin N, Popat R, Rismani A, et al. Whole-body MRI quantitative biomarkers are associated significantly with treatment response in patients with newly diagnosed symptomatic multiple myeloma following bortezomib induction. Eur Radiol. 2017;27(12):5325–36.
39. Messiou C, Kaiser M. Whole body diffusion weighted MRI–a new view of myeloma. Br J Haematol. 2015;171(1):29–37.
40. Horger M, Weisel K, Horger W, Mroue A, Fenchel M, Lichy M. Whole-body diffusion-weighted MRI with apparent diffusion coefficient mapping for early response monitoring in multiple myeloma: preliminary results. AJR Am J Roentgenol. 2011;196(6):W790–5.
41. Giles SL, Messiou C, Collins DJ, Morgan VA, Simpkin CJ, West S, et al. Whole-body diffusion-weighted MR imaging

for assessment of treatment response in myeloma. Radiology. 2014;271(3):785–94.
42. Wu C, Huang J, Xu W-B, Guan Y-J, Ling H-W, Mi J-Q, et al. Discriminating depth of response to therapy in multiple myeloma using whole-body diffusion-weighted MRI with apparent diffusion coefficient: preliminary results from a single-center study. Acad Radiol. *2018* 25(7):904–14.
43. Messiou C, Hillengass J, Delorme S, Lecouvet FE, Moulopoulos LA, Collins DJ, et al. Guidelines for acquisition, interpretation, and reporting of whole-body MRI in myeloma: Myeloma Response Assessment and Diagnosis System (MY-RADS). Radiology. 2019;291(1):5–13.
44. Moehler TM, Hawighorst H, Neben K, Egerer G, Hillengass J, Max R, et al. Bone marrow microcirculation analysis in multiple myeloma by contrast-enhanced dynamic magnetic resonance imaging. Int J Cancer. 2001;93(6):862–8.
45. Hose D, Moreaux J, Meissner T, Seckinger A, Goldschmidt H, Benner A, et al. Induction of angiogenesis by normal and malignant plasma cells. Blood. 2009;114(1):128–43.
46. Rajkumar SV, Leong T, Roche PC, Fonseca R, Dispenzieri A, Lacy MQ, et al. Prognostic value of bone marrow angiogenesis in multiple myeloma. Clin Cancer Res. 2000;6(8):3111–6.
47. Rajkumar SV, Mesa RA, Fonseca R, Schroeder G, Plevak MF, Dispenzieri A, et al. Bone marrow angiogenesis in 400 patients with monoclonal gammopathy of undetermined significance, multiple myeloma, and primary amyloidosis. Clin Cancer Res. 2002;8(7):2210–6.
48. Hillengass J, Zechmann C, Bäuerle T, Wagner-Gund B, Heiss C, Benner A, et al. Dynamic contrast-enhanced magnetic resonance imaging identifies a subgroup of patients with asymptomatic monoclonal plasma cell disease and pathologic microcirculation. Clin Cancer Res. 2009;15(9):3118–25.
49. Bhutani M, Turkbey B, Tan E, Kemp TJ, Pinto LA, Berg AR, et al. Bone marrow angiogenesis in myeloma and its precursor disease: a prospective clinical trial. Leukemia. 2014;28(2):413–6.
50. Merz M, Moehler TM, Ritsch J, Bäuerle T, Zechmann CM, Wagner B, et al. Prognostic significance of increased bone marrow microcirculation in newly diagnosed multiple myeloma: results of a prospective DCE-MRI study. Eur Radiol. 2016;26(5):1404–11.
51. Hillengass J, Ritsch J, Merz M, Wagner B, Kunz C, Hielscher T, et al. Increased microcirculation detected by dynamic contrast-enhanced magnetic resonance imaging is of prog-

nostic significance in asymptomatic myeloma. Br J Haematol. 2016;174(1):127–35.
52. Dutoit JC, Claus E, Offner F, Noens L, Delanghe J, Verstraete KL. Combined evaluation of conventional MRI, dynamic contrast-enhanced MRI and diffusion weighted imaging for response evaluation of patients with multiple myeloma. Eur J Radiol. 2016;85(2):373–82.
53. Terpos E, Matsaridis D, Koutoulidis V, Zagouri F, Christoulas D, Fontara S, et al. Dynamic contrast-enhanced magnetic resonance imaging parameters correlate with advanced revised-ISS and angiopoietin-1/angiopoietin-2 ratio in patients with multiple myeloma. Ann Hematol. 2017;96(10):1707–14.
54. Merz M, Ritsch J, Kunz C, Wagner B, Sauer S, Hose D, et al. Dynamic contrast-enhanced magnetic resonance imaging for assessment of antiangiogenic treatment effects in multiple myeloma. Clin Cancer Res. 2015;21(1):106–12.

Chapter 7
Therapy of Myeloma Bone Disease

Ioannis Ntanasis-Stathopoulos and Evangelos Terpos

Introduction

Bone disease affects up to 80% of the newly diagnosed patients with multiple myeloma (NDMM) [1]. These patients present with substantial bone pain, and they are at high risk for developing skeletal-related events (SREs), such as pathological fractures, spinal cord compression, and need for radiotherapeutic or surgical intervention [2]. Whole-body low-dose computed tomography is currently the new standard for evaluating myeloma bone disease (MBD) [3, 4]. Although there has been a substantial increase in overall survival (OS) in the past 10 years, over 80% of osteolytic lesions develop during management, underlining a key pitfall in controlling MBD [5–7]. MBD occurs due to the interaction between malignant plasma cells (MPCs) and cells in the bone marrow

---

I. Ntanasis-Stathopoulos · E. Terpos (✉)
Department of Clinical Therapeutics, Alexandra General Hospital, Medical School, National and Kapodistrian University of Athens, Athens, Greece
e-mail: eterpos@med.uoa.gr

E. Zamagni (ed.), *Management of Bone Disease and Kidney Failure in Multiple Myeloma*,
https://doi.org/10.1007/978-3-030-63662-3_7

microenvironment, leading to bone resorption and the formation of focal osteolytic lesions mediated by osteoclasts, and downregulation of the number of functional osteoblasts [8, 9]. MM cells interfere with physiologic bone remodeling by releasing osteoclast-promoting cytokines such as receptor activator of NF-kappa B ligand (RANKL), interleukin (IL)-1, IL-6, chemokine C-C motif ligand 3 (CCL3), and CLL20. More recently, activin-A has been implicated in MM bone disease, through stimulating RANK expression and inducing osteoclast genesis [10–12]. Moreover, Wnt signaling pathway inhibitors, such as dickkopf-1 (DKK-1) and sclerostin, are important inhibitors of osteoblast function [12, 13]. These enlarged insights into the pathophysiology improved the understanding of myeloma cell growth and bone destruction leading to enhanced bone directed therapies.

Regarding MBD therapeutics, there is a vivid interest in translating the complex underlying pathophysiology into effective targeted agents [9]. Therapeutic strategies, targeting the pathophysiologic interaction between MM cells, osteoclasts, and osteoblasts in the bone marrow microenvironment, are fundamental to delay the incidence of SREs and to prevent bone lesions. Bisphosphonates, both inhibiting osteoclasts and inducing MM cell apoptosis, are currently the gold standard for the treatment of MBD. Bisphosphonates reduce SREs, improve quality of life, and in parts increase progression-free survival and OS. However adverse side effects such as renal impairment, osteonecrosis of the jaw, and the unmet clinical need to reverse bone destruction, require the development of novel agents [14]. The recently approved RANKL inhibitor, denosumab, is another bone-modifying agent with promising anti-catabolic properties for the treatment of MBD [15]. Additionally, there has been an increased interest in elucidating the role of osteocytes in MBD and in developing new therapeutic strategies that target osteocyte function [16]. Sclerostin is currently considered the major mediator of the molecular osteocyte mechanisms of bone responses [17]. Given the numerous findings regarding the involvement of sclerostin in bone remodeling, humanized sclerostin antibodies have been developed.

Physiopathology of Myeloma Bone Disease

Deregulation of Osteocytes

Physiological bone remodeling is highly dependent on the fine-tuned interactions among the bone matrix, osteocytes, osteoclasts, osteoblasts, and immune cells [18]. MBD is characterized by significant deregulation in all these aspects; the ultimate effect is the increased osteoclast activity and suppressed osteoblast function leading to bone loss. Osteocytes play a major role in these pathways through the secretion of receptor activator of nuclear factor (NF)-κB ligand (RANKL), sclerostin, dickkopf-1, and other not very well-studied factors [19–21]. MM cells lead osteocytes to apoptosis in order to alter the bone marrow microenvironment and provide a pre-metastatic niche for the MM cells [22]. Indeed, MM patients have reduced number of viable osteocytes, which is associated with increased bone disease burden [23]. On the other hand, proteasome inhibitors, which have a positive effect on bone formation in MM, have been shown to restore osteocyte viability by reducing autophagy and apoptosis in MM patients [24].

Increased Osteoclast Activity

A cardinal signaling cascade regulating osteoclast maturation and activation is the RANK/RANKL pathway. RANK is a receptor of the tumor necrosis factor (TNF) superfamily, mainly expressed on the surface of osteoclasts precursors, produced by bone marrow stromal cells (BMSCs), osteoblasts, and activated T-lymphocytes [25]. RANK ligand (RANKL) is the associated cytokine, predominantly secreted by osteocytes, BMSC, and osteoblasts, for the latter both to a lesser extent. By binding to RANK on immature osteoblasts, RANKL induces their differentiation into mature cells. The receptor activator of NF-κB (RANK)/RANK ligand (RANKL) signaling pathway has been identified as a crucial regulatory system of bone remodeling. Osteoprotegerin (OPG) is a decoy receptor of the TNF superfamily, which also binds to RANKL [26]. OPG is secreted by osteoblasts and blocks the interaction of RANKL with RANK, thus inhibiting osteoclastogenesis [27, 28]. OPG expression is regulated by IL-1b, TNF-α, TGF-β, oestradiol, and 18b-oestriol. MM cells degrade OPG through the membrane syndecan-1 system [29]. MM cells induce osteocyte apoptosis via activation of Notch signaling, leading to high levels of RANKL. Additionally, interactions of MM cells with the BM microenvironment lead to upregulation of different cytokines (IL-1 and TNF-) and hormones (parathyroid hormone-related protein), which upregulated RANKL expression and decreased OPG expression, resulting in an increase of osteoclast activity and bone destruction [30]. These effects result in an increased RANKL-OPG ratio in the bone marrow microenvironment and favor the formation and activation of osteoclasts. Therefore, the increased RANKL-OPG ratio favors bone destruction, and importantly it impacts prognosis of NDMM patients [31]. A positive correlation is known between the incidence of osteolytic lesions and increasing serum RANKL levels [32]. Overall, levels of OPG and RANKL correlate with the activity of the MM, severity of MBD, and an impaired prognosis [31, 33, 34]. These data highlight the therapeutic relevance of targeting the RANKL-OPG axis in the development of novel therapy strategies in MBD.

Another aberrant pathway inducing osteoclast activity is the Notch signaling. Both members of the Notch family and their Jagged ligands are expressed in the membrane of MM cells, enabling homotypical and heterotypical interactions with the same or adjacent cells, respectively. The subsequently activated intracellular cascade ultimately results in the increase of RANKL production by MM cells. However, in myeloma microenvironment BMSCs and osteocytes remain the main sources of RANKL [35, 36]. Other factors favoring osteoclastogenesis and osteoclast-mediated bone loss include chemokines such as C-C motif ligand-3 (CCL-3), stromal cell-derived factor-1α (SDF-1α), osteopontin, interleukins, annexin II, members of the transforming growth factor-β (TGF-β) superfamily such as activin-A, and members of the TNF superfamily such as TNF-α and B cell-activating factor (BAFF) [37–44].

Suppressed Osteoblast Activity

Wingless-type (Wnt) or β-catenin pathway is a principal regulator of osteoblast differentiation and bone homeostasis [45]. Osteocytes and MM cells express Wnt antagonists, such as sclerostin, dickkopf-1, and soluble frizzled-related proteins, and suppress osteoblast activity [46, 47].

Sclerostin is an osteocyte product associated with abnormal bone remodeling; it impedes the activation of the canonical Wnt pathway and inhibits osteoblast maturation, impairs bone mineralization, and induces osteoblast apoptosis though the caspase cascade activation [17, 48]. Sclerostin is a 22-kDa glycoprotein encoded by the SOST gene. It is mainly synthesized by different mature osteocytes, binds to Wnt co-receptors LRP5/6, and antagonizes the pathway [49]. Clinical studies showed that increased circulating sclerostin levels are evident in patients with active MM disease, which correlates with the presence of osteolytic fractures, abnormal bone remodeling, and disease stage [48]. Sclerostin inhibition with monoclonal antibodies in preclinical MM models restores the deregulated bone metabolism and decreases bone fragility [47, 50].

Dickkopf-1 has a synergistic effect with sclerostin and disrupts the autocrine Wnt signaling and, subsequently, suppresses osteoblast differentiation and activity [46, 51]. DKK-1 is expressed by osteoblasts and BMSCs and secreted by MM cells and antagonizes the Wnt pathway. Members of DKK-1 bind to lipoprotein receptor-related protein (LRP)-5/6, thus inhibiting osteoblastogenesis and new bone formation. DKK-1 is responsible for an increased sclerostin secretion in the bone microenvironment. In the presence of MM-derived DKK-1, sclerostin is released by immature osteoblasts [52]. In

MM patients, gene expression levels and serum levels of DKK-1 correlate with the extent of MBD [51, 53]; as a result, mesenchymal stem cells do not differentiate to osteoblasts [51]. Since the Wnt signaling pathway in osteoclasts increases the expression of OPG and downregulates the expression of RANKL, inhibition of Wnt signaling pathway promotes osteoclastogenesis [54, 55].

Other regulatory factors of the Wnt pathway that are found deregulated in MM include periostin, runt-related transcription factor 2, and growth factor independence-1 [56–58]. Furthermore, members of the TGF-β and TNF superfamilies along with interleukins are also implicated in favoring osteoblast suppression, while osteoclasts and myeloma cells further inhibit osteoblasts through semaphorin-4D [59–61]. Interestingly, proteasome inhibitors promote osteoblast differentiation by upregulating the intracellular beta-catenin pathway independently of Wnt signaling; thus they have an anabolic effect on myelomatous bone [22, 62, 63].

Bone Marrow Microenvironment

In the bone marrow microenvironment, there is a constant crosstalk among the different cell subtypes [64]. Homing of MM cells is favored by their adhesion to BMSCs through the VLA-4/VCAM-1 integrin system [65]. Notch bidirectional signaling also mediates interactions among MM cells, BMSCs, and osteocytes and leads to significant alterations in bone marrow microenvironment promoting MM proliferation and bone destruction [35, 36]. The deregulated EphrinB2/EphB4 signaling in MM also impairs the normal interaction between osteoclasts and osteoblasts, which finally results in increased bone loss [66]. Osteoclasts potentiate the immunosuppressive microenvironment by promoting the expansion of Th17 lymphocytes and myeloid-derived suppressor cells, whereas they inhibit the cytotoxic T- and NK-cells against MM cells [67, 68]. The upregulation of immune checkpoint molecules and T-cell metabolism regulators provide the rationale for targeted monoclonal antibodies against programmed death ligand 1 and CD38 [68, 69]. Interestingly, the interplay between MM cells and mature osteoblasts may provide a unique niche for MM cells to be maintained in quiescence, whereas osteoblast dysfunction or osteoclast remodeling of the endosteal niche allows their reactivation [70–72].

Treatment of Myeloma Bone Disease

An overview of major randomized clinical trials on bone-targeting agents for the treatment of MBD is provided in Table 7.1 [15, 73–78].

Bisphosphonates

Bisphosphonates remain the cornerstone for the management of myeloma-related bone disease. Bisphosphonates are pyrophosphate analogues that bind to exposed bone areas of hydroxyapatite crystals. During bone remodeling, they are absorbed by the osteoclasts, and they inhibit intracellular farnesyl pyrophosphate synthase; thus, bisphosphonates impair osteoclastogenesis and disrupt osteoclast activity [79].

Three major "head-to-head" randomized studies of the most effective bisphosphonates on MBD has been performed. In a randomized phase II trial, escalating intravenous doses (0.4 mg–4.0 mg) of zoledronic acid were compared with 90 mg intravenous pamidronate in MM or metastatic breast cancer patients [73]. In terms of pain reduction and SRE, zoledronic acid (administered 2 or 4 mg/months) proved to be as effective as 90 mg pamidronate, with greater doses of zoledronic acid reduced the need of radiation.

A large phase III, randomized, double-blind trial compared pamidronate with zoledronic acid in 1648 patients with MM Durie-Salmon stage III or advanced breast cancer with bone lesions [74]. Although no difference in time to the first SRE between the two therapy groups became evident, skel-

Table 7.1 Summary of major randomized clinical trials on bone-targeting agents for the treatment of MBD [96]

Study	Treatment drug	Treatment schedule	Number of patients	Median time to first SRE (months)	SRE incidence	ONJ	Renal toxicity
Berenson et al. [73]	Pamidronate vs Placebo	Pamidronate 90 mg every 4 weeks for 9 cycles	196 vs. 181	Shorter in the placebo group ($p = 0.001$)	24% vs. 41% ($p < 0.001$)	NR	NR
Rosen et al. [74]	Zoledronic acid vs. pamidronate	4 or 8 mg of zoledronic acid i.v. or 90 mg of i.v. pamidronate every 3–4 weeks for 12 months	129 vs. 65	12.5 vs. 9.4	NR	NR	NR
Gimsing et al. [75]	Pamidronate	Pamidronate 30 mg vs. pamidronate 90 mg	252 vs. 252	10.2 vs. 9.2 ($p = 0.63$)	33.7% vs. 35.2%	0.8% vs. 3.2%	NR

Morgan et al. [76, 77]	Zoledronic acid vs. clodronate	4 mg zoledronic acid i.v. every 3–4 weeks or 1600 mg oral clodronic acid daily	981 vs. 979	NR	27% vs. 35% ($p = 0.0004$)	4% vs. <1%	Similar for the two treatment groups ($p = 0.55$)
Himelstein et al. [78]	Zoledronic acid	Zoledronic acid every 12 vs. every 4 weeks	139 vs. 139	NR	55% vs. 60%	NR	NR
Raje et al. [15]	Denosumab vs. zoledronic acid	s.c. denosumab 120 mg plus i.v. placebo or i.v. zoledronic acid 4 mg plus s.c. placebo every 4 weeks	859 vs. 859	22.8 vs. 24 ($p_{non\text{-}inferiority} = 0.01$)	43.8% vs. 44.6%	4.1% vs. 2.8%	10% vs. 17.1%

SRE skeletal-related events, *ONJ* osteonecrosis of the jaw, *PFS* progression-free survival, *OS* overall survival, *NR* not reported, *s.c.* subcutaneous, *i.v.* intravenous etal morbidity rate was minimally increased in patients treated with pamidronate. However, the incidence of radiation therapy significantly increased in patients treated with pamidronate compared to zoledronic acid.

The Myeloma IX trial, conducted by the Medical Research Council (MRC), a multi-center randomized, open-label study, compared the effect of oral clodronate (1600 mg/day) versus i.v. zoledronate (4 mg i.v. every 21–28 days, dose adjusted based on creatinine clearance levels) for patients with NDMM [76]. According to the MRC trial, patients treated with zoledronic acid revealed fewer on study SREs: after a median follow-up of 3.7 years, 27% of patients receiving zoledronic acid had experienced SREs versus 35% receiving clodronate ($p = 0.004$). Moreover, zoledronic acid was associated with a reduced risk of mortality (HR 0.84; $p = 0.0118$) with an extended median overall survival of 5.5 months (50 months vs. 44.5 months; $p = 0.04$) and an increased median progression-free survival of 2 months (19.5 months vs. 17.5 months; $p = 0.07$). This benefit could not be explained by the favorable effect on SREs alone. More importantly, these observations confirm preclinical studies that zoledronic acid may have direct or indirect anti-myeloma effect in addition to its antiresorptive effects [80].

An updated meta-analysis including 7293 patients has tried to provide a comparative evaluation among the currently available bisphosphonates [81]. Although all agents showed substantial efficacy in reducing SREs and bone pain, none of the approved bisphosphonates (clodronate, pamidronate, or zoledronic acid) showed superiority over another in any of the outcomes [81]. Interestingly, zoledronic acid provided a survival advantage. The Myeloma IX trial showed that zoledronic acid increased median OS as compared to clodronate [76]. Zoledronic acid may exert direct anti-myeloma effects by inhibition of protein prenylation or indirect through downregulating BMSC-related adhesion molecules and blocking osteoclast activation [79, 82, 83].

Despite bisphosphonates being the initial choice of treatment, the durability of their use is limited to their side effects. The main side effects of bisphosphonates are renal toxicity and osteonecrosis of the jaw (ONJ); thus, close monitoring of patients undergoing long-term treatment of bisphosphonates is warranted. Up to 40% of bisphosphonates were excreted via glomerular filtration and active tubular excretion [84]; therefore kidneys play a cornerstone within the adverse side effects of bisphosphonates. While pamidronate induces rather glomerular damage, zoledronate revealed to induce acute tubular necrosis, both potentially resulting in acute renal failure [85]. The nephrotoxicity correlates with dose, time of infusion, and maximum plasma concentration. Zoledronic acid doses should be reduced in patients with creatinine levels of 30–60 ml/min. Although studies of zoledronic acid in patients with severe renal impairment have not been performed, there is no recommendation in these patient cohorts. In contrast, pamidronate (90 mg administered over 4–6 h) is recommended in patients with severe renal impairment [86]. Rare complications during the long-term therapy with bisphosphonates are atypical femoral fractures, occurring with minimal trauma [87], increased risk of congestive heart failure, and atrial fibrillation, especially in patients with osteoporosis using nitrogen-containing bisphosphonates [88, 89].

The optimal use of bisphosphonates in MM patients is continuously under investigation taking into account the potential side effects. The International Myeloma Working group (IMWG) recommends that bisphosphonates should be given until disease progression in MM patients without achieving complete response or very good partial response [90]. Additionally, bone marker-guided administration of bisphosphonates was evaluated in the recent Zoledronic-Acid-Bone MARKer-Directed Dosing (Z-MARK) and demonstrated that less-frequent zoledronic acid administration (every 12 weeks >2 years) was not associated with higher increase of SREs (5.8% SREs within the first year vs. 4.9% in the second year) [75].

Denosumab

Denosumab is a fully human, monoclonal antibody of IgG2 class that binds to RANKL with high specificity and prevents its interaction with RANK; thus, it mimics the effect of endogenous OPG and inhibits bone resorption [91]. Denosumab binds only to RANKL and not to other members of the TNF family, such as TNF-α, TNF-β, TNF-related apoptosis-inducing ligand, and CD40 ligand, therefore providing a high affinity and specificity [92]. Until early 2018, denosumab was licensed for postmenopausal women with osteoporosis and patients with either primary giant cell tumors of the bone or bone metastases secondary to solid tumors. In 2018, both FDA and EMA granted supplemental approval for denosumab for the prevention of SREs among MM patients based on the results of the 20090482 phase 3 study [15].

In a phase II trial, Vij et al. analyzed the efficacy of denosumab in MM patients with relapsed or plateau phase of their disease [93]. Denosumab, when administered monthly at a dose of 120 mg s.c. (with additional loading doses on day 8 and 15 within the first months), effectively inhibited the RANKL pathway, expressed by a decreased serum C-terminal cross-linking telopeptide of collagen type 1 (CTX) level more than 50%, irrespective of the previous exposure of patients to bisphosphonates. Interestingly, in 80% of the patients, denosumab was discontinued due to disease progression and absence of complete or partial response. These data strongly warranted to analyze the efficacy of denosumab according to the ability to prevent SREs in further clinical trials. Fizazi et al. analyzed in a phase II in vivo study patients with MM or prostate or breast cancer who were initially treated with bisphosphonates and were randomized to receive either denosumab every 4 or 12 weeks. The trial showed that denosumab was able to suppress the bone turnover and decrease the incidence of SREs in patients who were initially treated with bisphosphonates compared to the i.v. bisphosphonates therapy group (8% vs. 17%, respectively) [94].

The 20090482 phase 3 study was an international, double-blind, double-dummy, 1:1 randomized controlled trial that evaluated the efficacy and safety of denosumab compared to zoledronic acid among 1718 NDMM patients [15]. After a median time on study of 17.3 and 17.6 months for denosumab and zoledronic acid group, respectively, denosumab was non-inferior to zoledronic acid in delaying time to first SRE, which was the primary study endpoint (HR 0.98, 95% CI: 0.85–1.14; $p_{\text{non-inferiority}} = 0.010$). Interestingly, a post hoc landmark analysis at 15 months suggested denosumab superiority for time to first SRE (HR 0.66, 95% CI: 0.44–0.98; $p = 0.039$). Although the data were rather immature to reach firm conclusions on the secondary endpoint of OS, denosumab demonstrated a clinically meaningful median PFS benefit of 10.7 months ($p = 0.036$) compared to zoledronic acid on top of standard of care first-line anti-myeloma treatment [15]. A supplemental analysis according to pre-specified patient subgroups on the latter exploratory endpoint has been recently provided. It seems that the PFS impact of denosumab is more pronounced among NDMM patients receiving first-line therapy based on proteasome inhibitors without immunomodulatory drugs ($p = 0.019$) and those who received an autologous stem cell transplant ($p = 0.002$) [95].

Denosumab is administered subcutaneously at 120 mg every 4 weeks in NDMM patients [15]. Currently, there is an open debate on whether and under what circumstances could denosumab treatment be discontinued [96]. Due to lack of pertinent data on solid malignancies and MM, there are recommendations based on osteoporosis studies. In contrast to bisphosphonates, denosumab is not incorporated into the bone matrix and does not show prolonged effects after its discontinuation [97]. Denosumab cessation leads to reduced bone mineral density and increased risk of fractures after 12–18 months post its discontinuation [97]. Therefore, bridging with antiresorptive agents (i.e., one dose of i.v. bisphosphonate) is considered vital among patients who discontinue denosumab in order to preserve the attained favorable effect on bone indices in post-menopausal osteoporosis patients

[98]. Studies on this topic are urgently needed in order to provide specific recommendations for MM patients.

Denosumab is generally well tolerated, and some side effects associated with zoledronic acid are less common or not reported with denosumab. Unlike bisphosphonates, denosumab does not accumulate in the bone. In accordance with other monoclonal antibodies, the clearance of denosumab does not depend on renal function [99]. Previous phase III studies observed less frequently renal dysfunction with denosumab compared to zoledronic acid in patients with metastatic bone disease [100]. Raje et al. confirmed these results in MM patients and demonstrated significant differences between denosumab and zoledronic acid in terms of renal toxicity [15]. In patients with baseline creatinine clearance ≤60 ml/min, denosumab revealed less renal toxicity compared to zoledronic acid (13% vs. 26%; $p < 0.01$), and doubled serum creatinine from baseline was nearly twice high in the zoledronic acid arm (7% vs. 3.3%).

ONJ is a serious complication of therapy with targeting osteoclast, and it was first reported with i.v. bisphosphonates in the early 2000s. While the risk of ONJ has also been observed with denosumab therapy primarily in patients with solid tumors and bone metastases [101, 102], similar incidence between denosumab and zoledronic acid (4% vs. 3%, respectively, $p = 0.147$) was observed in MM patients [15].

Hypocalcemia was more frequent in the denosumab (17%) than the zoledronic acid (12%) group in the 20,090,482 trial [15]. Serum calcium, vitamin D, phosphate, and magnesium should be evaluated on a regular basis to assess the need for additional supplementation in patients with MM receiving bone-targeted agents [90].

Anti-sclerostin Antibodies

Besides an inhibition of osteoclastic resorption, a comprehensive therapy of MBD in MM patients requires also a stimulation of osteoblastic bone formation. A superior preventive strategy is to target osteocytes in the bone microenvironment, and in recent years, sclerostin, a Wnt/β-catenin inhibitor that controls bone formation, is of growing interest to elucidate the role of osteocytes in MBD.

Neutralizing antibodies such as the humanized monoclonal anti-sclerostin antibodies romosozumab and blosozumab have been already evaluated in the clinical setting in patients with osteoporosis [103] and are considered potential agents for MBD [104]. A randomized, double-blind trial was performed in healthy men and postmenopausal women receiving s.c. or i.v. romosozumab vs. placebo [105]. The results revealed that romosozumab increased serum levels of bone formation markers such as P1NP or bone-specific alkaline phosphatase (BSAP) and decreased bone resorption of CTX in comparison to placebo [105]. These results were translated in a significant improvement of vertebral trabecular and cortical bone, lasting over the follow-up period of given administration [104, 106].

Since sclerostin inhibition alone has no significant anti-MM activity [50], therapeutic strategies aim to combine sclerostin antibodies and anti-MM agents. Recent in vitro treatment of MM cells with anti-sclerostin antibodies in combination with anti-MM agents, such as bortezomib and dexamethasone, did not provide any anti-MM activity, promoting to investigate the use for additional combination therapies [52]. More recently, effects of anti-sclerostin antibody alone and in combination with bisphosphonate therapy on the skeleton in a series of well-characterized murine and human xenograft models of myeloma bone disease have been tested [50]. McDonald et al. showed that anti-sclerostin antibody alone and zoledronic acid alone both prevented myeloma-induced bone loss and that anti-sclerostin antibody alone increased bone strength. Moreover, results could highlight that anti-sclerostin antibody was superior to zoledronic at improving bone strength. Treatment by adding anti-sclerostin antibody to zoledronic acid increased bone volume over treatment and resistance to fracture when compared with zoledronic acid alone. These findings suggest that the combination of anti-sclerostin antibody and zoledronic acid therapy will offer additive clinically relevant benefits compared to the current standard of MBD [50]. This theoretical rationale has to be translated into clinical benefit in upcoming clinical trials.

Conclusion

Although bisphosphonates have been the mainstay of MBD for several years, denosumab may be an acceptable, cost-effective alternative considering its non-inferiority in terms of SRE prevention and the potential to minimize renal toxicity and improve PFS [107]. A further understanding of MBD biology may be translated into novel combinations of anti-myeloma and bone-targeting agents that would both reduce disease burden and restore bone metabolism. Anti-sclerostin agents seem to be the more promising to enter in clinical development for MM and potentially enhance our armamentarium of bone-targeted agents against MBD.

Acknowledgements None

Conflict of Interest Disclosure

ET has received honoraria from Amgen, Celgene, Genesis, Janssen, Novartis, BMS, and Takeda; is a member of SC for Amgen and Takeda and a member of IDMC for Celgene; and has received research grants from Amgen, Janssen, and Takeda. INS has no relevant conflict of interest.

References

1. Kyle RA, Gertz MA, Witzig TE, Lust JA, Lacy MQ, Dispenzieri A, et al. Review of 1027 patients with newly diagnosed multiple myeloma. Mayo Clin Proc. 2003;78(1):21–33.
2. Terpos E, Berenson J, Cook RJ, Lipton A, Coleman RE. Prognostic variables for survival and skeletal complications in patients with multiple myeloma osteolytic bone disease. Leukemia. 2010;24(5):1043–9.

3. Hillengass J, Moulopoulos LA, Delorme S, Koutoulidis V, Mosebach J, Hielscher T, et al. Whole-body computed tomography versus conventional skeletal survey in patients with multiple myeloma: a study of the International Myeloma Working Group. Blood Cancer J 2017;7(8):e599.
4. Moulopoulos LA, Koutoulidis V, Hillengass J, Zamagni E, Aquerreta JD, Roche CL, et al. Recommendations for acquisition, interpretation and reporting of whole body low dose CT in patients with multiple myeloma and other plasma cell disorders: a report of the IMWG Bone Working Group. Blood Cancer J. 2018;8(10):95.
5. Kumar SK, Dispenzieri A, Lacy MQ, Gertz MA, Buadi FK, Pandey S, et al. Continued improvement in survival in multiple myeloma: changes in early mortality and outcomes in older patients. Leukemia. 2014;28(5):1122–8.
6. Walker RE, Lawson MA, Buckle CH, Snowden JA, Chantry AD. Myeloma bone disease: pathogenesis, current treatments and future targets. Br Med Bull. 2014;111(1):117–38.
7. Engelhardt M, Terpos E, Kleber M, Gay F, Wasch R, Morgan G, et al. European Myeloma Network recommendations on the evaluation and treatment of newly diagnosed patients with multiple myeloma. Haematologica. 2014;99(2):232–42.
8. Roodman GD. Mechanisms of bone metastasis. N Engl J Med. 2004;350(16):1655–64.
9. Terpos E, Ntanasis-Stathopoulos I, Gavriatopoulou M, Dimopoulos MA. Pathogenesis of bone disease in multiple myeloma: from bench to bedside. Blood Cancer J. 2018;8(1):7.
10. Sugatani T, Alvarez UM, Hruska KA. Activin A stimulates IkappaB-alpha/NFkappaB and RANK expression for osteoclast differentiation, but not AKT survival pathway in osteoclast precursors. J Cell Biochem. 2003;90(1):59–67.
11. Yasuda H, Shima N, Nakagawa N, Yamaguchi K, Kinosaki M, Mochizuki S, et al. Osteoclast differentiation factor is a ligand for osteoprotegerin/osteoclastogenesis-inhibitory factor and is identical to TRANCE/RANKL. Proc Natl Acad Sci U S A. 1998;95(7):3597–602.
12. Gavriatopoulou M, Dimopoulos MA, Christoulas D, Migkou M, Iakovaki M, Gkotzamanidou M, et al. Dickkopf-1: a suitable target for the management of myeloma bone disease. Expert Opin Ther Targets. 2009;13(7):839–48.
13. Moester MJ, Papapoulos SE, Lowik CW, van Bezooijen RL. Sclerostin: current knowledge and future perspectives. Calcif Tissue Int. 2010;87(2):99–107.

14. Terpos E, Roodman GD, Dimopoulos MA. Optimal use of bisphosphonates in patients with multiple myeloma. Blood. 2013;121(17):3325–8.
15. Raje N, Terpos E, Willenbacher W, Shimizu K, Garcia-Sanz R, Durie B, et al. Denosumab versus zoledronic acid in bone disease treatment of newly diagnosed multiple myeloma: an international, double-blind, double-dummy, randomised, controlled, phase 3 study. Lancet Oncol. 2018;19(3):370–81.
16. Delgado-Calle J, Bellido T, Roodman GD. Role of osteocytes in multiple myeloma bone disease. Curr Opin Support Palliat Care. 2014;8(4):407–13.
17. Colucci S, Brunetti G, Oranger A, Mori G, Sardone F, Specchia G, et al. Myeloma cells suppress osteoblasts through sclerostin secretion. Blood Cancer J. 2011;1(6):e27.
18. Xiao W, Wang Y, Pacios S, Li S, Graves DT. Cellular and molecular aspects of bone remodeling. Front Oral Biol. 2016;18:9–16.
19. Nakashima T, Hayashi M, Fukunaga T, Kurata K, Oh-Hora M, Feng JQ, et al. Evidence for osteocyte regulation of bone homeostasis through RANKL expression. Nat Med. 2011;17(10):1231–4.
20. Poole KE, van Bezooijen RL, Loveridge N, Hamersma H, Papapoulos SE, Lowik CW, et al. Sclerostin is a delayed secreted product of osteocytes that inhibits bone formation. FASEB J. 2005;19(13):1842–4.
21. Li J, Sarosi I, Cattley RC, Pretorius J, Asuncion F, Grisanti M, et al. Dkk1-mediated inhibition of Wnt signaling in bone results in osteopenia. Bone. 2006;39(4):754–66.
22. Qiang YW, Hu B, Chen Y, Zhong Y, Shi B, Barlogie B, et al. Bortezomib induces osteoblast differentiation via Wnt-independent activation of beta-catenin/TCF signaling. Blood. 2009;113(18):4319–30.
23. Giuliani N, Ferretti M, Bolzoni M, Storti P, Lazzaretti M, Dalla Palma B, et al. Increased osteocyte death in multiple myeloma patients: role in myeloma-induced osteoclast formation. Leukemia. 2012;26(6):1391–401.
24. Toscani D, Palumbo C, Dalla Palma B, Ferretti M, Bolzoni M, Marchica V, et al. The proteasome inhibitor bortezomib maintains osteocyte viability in multiple myeloma patients by reducing both apoptosis and autophagy: a new function for proteasome inhibitors. J Bone Miner Res. 2016;31(4):815–27.
25. Hsu H, Lacey DL, Dunstan CR, Solovyev I, Colombero A, Timms E, et al. Tumor necrosis factor receptor family mem-

ber RANK mediates osteoclast differentiation and activation induced by osteoprotegerin ligand. Proc Natl Acad Sci U S A. 1999;96(7):3540–5.
26. Lacey DL, Timms E, Tan HL, Kelley MJ, Dunstan CR, Burgess T, et al. Osteoprotegerin ligand is a cytokine that regulates osteoclast differentiation and activation. Cell. 1998;93(2):165–76.
27. Boyle WJ, Simonet WS, Lacey DL. Osteoclast differentiation and activation. Nature. 2003;423(6937):337–42.
28. Mulcahy LE, Taylor D, Lee TC, Duffy GP. RANKL and OPG activity is regulated by injury size in networks of osteocyte-like cells. Bone. 2011;48(2):182–8.
29. Standal T, Seidel C, Hjertner O, Plesner T, Sanderson RD, Waage A, et al. Osteoprotegerin is bound, internalized, and degraded by multiple myeloma cells. Blood. 2002;100(8):3002–7.
30. Pearse RN, Sordillo EM, Yaccoby S, Wong BR, Liau DF, Colman N, et al. Multiple myeloma disrupts the TRANCE/osteoprotegerin cytokine axis to trigger bone destruction and promote tumor progression. Proc Natl Acad Sci U S A. 2001;98(20):11581–6.
31. Terpos E, Szydlo R, Apperley JF, Hatjiharissi E, Politou M, Meletis J, et al. Soluble receptor activator of nuclear factor kappaB ligand-osteoprotegerin ratio predicts survival in multiple myeloma: proposal for a novel prognostic index. Blood. 2003;102(3):1064–9.
32. Heider U, Langelotz C, Jakob C, Zavrski I, Fleissner C, Eucker J, et al. Expression of receptor activator of nuclear factor kappaB ligand on bone marrow plasma cells correlates with osteolytic bone disease in patients with multiple myeloma. Clin Cancer Res. 2003;9(4):1436–40.
33. Terpos E, Politou M, Szydlo R, Goldman JM, Apperley JF, Rahemtulla A. Serum levels of macrophage inflammatory protein-1 alpha (MIP-1alpha) correlate with the extent of bone disease and survival in patients with multiple myeloma. Br J Haematol. 2003;123(1):106–9.
34. Politou M, Terpos E, Anagnostopoulos A, Szydlo R, Laffan M, Layton M, et al. Role of receptor activator of nuclear factor-kappa B ligand (RANKL), osteoprotegerin and macrophage protein 1-alpha (MIP-1a) in monoclonal gammopathy of undetermined significance (MGUS). Br J Haematol. 2004;126(5):686–9.
35. Colombo M, Mirandola L, Platonova N, Apicella L, Basile A, Figueroa AJ, et al. Notch-directed microenvironment repro-

gramming in myeloma: a single path to multiple outcomes. Leukemia. 2013;27(5):1009–18.
36. Delgado-Calle J, Anderson J, Cregor MD, Hiasa M, Chirgwin JM, Carlesso N, et al. Bidirectional notch signaling and osteocyte-derived factors in the bone marrow microenvironment promote tumor cell proliferation and bone destruction in multiple myeloma. Cancer Res. 2016;76(5):1089–100.
37. Terpos E, Heath DJ, Rahemtulla A, Zervas K, Chantry A, Anagnostopoulos A, et al. Bortezomib reduces serum dickkopf-1 and receptor activator of nuclear factor-kappaB ligand concentrations and normalises indices of bone remodelling in patients with relapsed multiple myeloma. Br J Haematol. 2006;135(5):688–92.
38. Roussou M, Tasidou A, Dimopoulos MA, Kastritis E, Migkou M, Christoulas D, et al. Increased expression of macrophage inflammatory protein-1alpha on trephine biopsies correlates with extensive bone disease, increased angiogenesis and advanced stage in newly diagnosed patients with multiple myeloma. Leukemia. 2009;23(11):2177–81.
39. Terpos E, Kastritis E, Christoulas D, Gkotzamanidou M, Eleutherakis-Papaiakovou E, Kanellias N, et al. Circulating activin-A is elevated in patients with advanced multiple myeloma and correlates with extensive bone involvement and inferior survival; no alterations post-lenalidomide and dexamethasone therapy. Ann Oncol. 2012;23(10):2681–6.
40. Vallet S, Mukherjee S, Vaghela N, Hideshima T, Fulciniti M, Pozzi S, et al. Activin A promotes multiple myeloma-induced osteolysis and is a promising target for myeloma bone disease. Proc Natl Acad Sci U S A. 2010;107(11):5124–9.
41. Lee JW, Chung HY, Ehrlich LA, Jelinek DF, Callander NS, Roodman GD, et al. IL-3 expression by myeloma cells increases both osteoclast formation and growth of myeloma cells. Blood. 2004;103(6):2308–15.
42. Noonan K, Marchionni L, Anderson J, Pardoll D, Roodman GD, Borrello I. A novel role of IL-17-producing lymphocytes in mediating lytic bone disease in multiple myeloma. Blood. 2010;116(18):3554–63.
43. Hengeveld PJ, Kersten MJ. B-cell activating factor in the pathophysiology of multiple myeloma: a target for therapy? Blood Cancer J. 2015;5:e282.
44. Wang XT, He YC, Zhou SY, Jiang JZ, Huang YM, Liang YZ, et al. Bone marrow plasma macrophage inflammatory pro-

tein protein-1 alpha(MIP-1 alpha) and sclerostin in multiple myeloma: relationship with bone disease and clinical characteristics. Leuk Res. 2014;38(5):525–31.
45. Baron R, Kneissel M. WNT signaling in bone homeostasis and disease: from human mutations to treatments. Nat Med. 2013;19(2):179–92.
46. Qiang YW, Chen Y, Stephens O, Brown N, Chen B, Epstein J, et al. Myeloma-derived Dickkopf-1 disrupts Wnt-regulated osteoprotegerin and RANKL production by osteoblasts: a potential mechanism underlying osteolytic bone lesions in multiple myeloma. Blood. 2008;112(1):196–207.
47. Delgado-Calle J, Anderson J, Cregor MD, Condon KW, Kuhstoss SA, Plotkin LI, et al. Genetic deletion of Sost or pharmacological inhibition of sclerostin prevent multiple myeloma-induced bone disease without affecting tumor growth. Leukemia. 2017;31(12):2686–94.
48. Terpos E, Christoulas D, Katodritou E, Bratengeier C, Gkotzamanidou M, Michalis E, et al. Elevated circulating sclerostin correlates with advanced disease features and abnormal bone remodeling in symptomatic myeloma: reduction post-bortezomib monotherapy. Int J Cancer. 2012;131(6):1466–71.
49. Delgado-Calle J, Sato AY, Bellido T. Role and mechanism of action of sclerostin in bone. Bone. 2017;96:29–37.
50. McDonald MM, Reagan MR, Youlten SE, Mohanty ST, Seckinger A, Terry RL, et al. Inhibiting the osteocyte-specific protein sclerostin increases bone mass and fracture resistance in multiple myeloma. Blood. 2017;129(26):3452–64.
51. Tian E, Zhan F, Walker R, Rasmussen E, Ma Y, Barlogie B, et al. The role of the Wnt-signaling antagonist DKK1 in the development of osteolytic lesions in multiple myeloma. N Engl J Med. 2003;349(26):2483–94.
52. Eda H, Santo L, Wein MN, Hu DZ, Cirstea DD, Nemani N, et al. Regulation of sclerostin expression in multiple myeloma by Dkk-1: a potential therapeutic strategy for myeloma Bone disease. J Bone Miner Res. 2016;31(6):1225–34.
53. Kaiser M, Mieth M, Liebisch P, Oberlander R, Rademacher J, Jakob C, et al. Serum concentrations of DKK-1 correlate with the extent of bone disease in patients with multiple myeloma. Eur J Haematol. 2008;80(6):490–4.
54. Spencer GJ, Utting JC, Etheridge SL, Arnett TR, Genever PG. Wnt signalling in osteoblasts regulates expression of the

receptor activator of NFkappaB ligand and inhibits osteoclastogenesis in vitro. J Cell Sci. 2006;119(Pt 7):1283–96.
55. Glass DA 2nd, Bialek P, Ahn JD, Starbuck M, Patel MS, Clevers H, et al. Canonical Wnt signaling in differentiated osteoblasts controls osteoclast differentiation. Dev Cell. 2005;8(5):751–64.
56. Terpos E, Christoulas D, Kastritis E, Bagratuni T, Gavriatopoulou M, Roussou M, et al. High levels of periostin correlate with increased fracture rate, diffuse MRI pattern, abnormal bone remodeling and advanced disease stage in patients with newly diagnosed symptomatic multiple myeloma. Blood Cancer J. 2016;6(10):e482.
57. Giuliani N, Colla S, Morandi F, Lazzaretti M, Sala R, Bonomini S, et al. Myeloma cells block RUNX2/CBFA1 activity in human bone marrow osteoblast progenitors and inhibit osteoblast formation and differentiation. Blood. 2005;106(7):2472–83.
58. D'Souza S, del Prete D, Jin S, Sun Q, Huston AJ, Kostov FE, et al. Gfi1 expressed in bone marrow stromal cells is a novel osteoblast suppressor in patients with multiple myeloma bone disease. Blood. 2011;118(26):6871–80.
59. Negishi-Koga T, Shinohara M, Komatsu N, Bito H, Kodama T, Friedel RH, et al. Suppression of bone formation by osteoclastic expression of semaphorin 4D. Nat Med. 2011;17(11):1473–80.
60. Takeuchi K, Abe M, Hiasa M, Oda A, Amou H, Kido S, et al. Tgf-Beta inhibition restores terminal osteoblast differentiation to suppress myeloma growth. PLoS One. 2010;5(3):e9870.
61. Terpos E, Ntanasis-Stathopoulos I, Christoulas D, Bagratuni T, Bakogeorgos M, Gavriatopoulou M, et al. Semaphorin 4D correlates with increased bone resorption, hypercalcemia, and disease stage in newly diagnosed patients with multiple myeloma. Blood Cancer J. 2018;8(5):42.
62. Hu B, Chen Y, Usmani SZ, Ye S, Qiang W, Papanikolaou X, et al. Characterization of the molecular mechanism of the bone-anabolic activity of carfilzomib in multiple myeloma. PLoS One. 2013;8(9):e74191.
63. Garcia-Gomez A, Quwaider D, Canavese M, Ocio EM, Tian Z, Blanco JF, et al. Preclinical activity of the oral proteasome inhibitor MLN9708 in Myeloma bone disease. Clin Cancer Res. 2014;20(6):1542–54.
64. Mondello P, Cuzzocrea S, Navarra M, Mian M. Bone marrow micro-environment is a crucial player for myelomagenesis and disease progression. Oncotarget. 2017;8(12):20394–409.

65. Mori Y, Shimizu N, Dallas M, Niewolna M, Story B, Williams PJ, et al. Anti-alpha4 integrin antibody suppresses the development of multiple myeloma and associated osteoclastic osteolysis. Blood. 2004;104(7):2149–54.
66. Pennisi A, Ling W, Li X, Khan S, Shaughnessy JD Jr, Barlogie B, et al. The ephrinB2/EphB4 axis is dysregulated in osteoprogenitors from myeloma patients and its activation affects myeloma bone disease and tumor growth. Blood. 2009;114(9):1803–12.
67. Mukaihara K, Siu K, Panaroni C, Fulzele K, Soucy R, Huang C, et al. The pleiotropic immunosuppressive role of osteoclasts in multiple myeloma. Blood. 2018;132:4447.
68. An G, Acharya C, Feng X, Wen K, Zhong M, Zhang L, et al. Osteoclasts promote immune suppressive microenvironment in multiple myeloma: therapeutic implication. Blood. 2016;128(12):1590–603.
69. Costa F, Toscani D, Chillemi A, Quarona V, Bolzoni M, Marchica V, et al. Expression of CD38 in myeloma bone niche: a rational basis for the use of anti-CD38 immunotherapy to inhibit osteoclast formation. Oncotarget. 2017;8(34):56598–611.
70. Fulzele K, Panaroni C, Soucy R, Siu K, Mukaihara K, Raje N. Mature osteoblasts provide a protective niche against multiple myeloma growth and survival within the tumor microenvironment. Blood. 2018;132:4476.
71. Chen Z, Orlowski RZ, Wang M, Kwak L, McCarty N. Osteoblastic niche supports the growth of quiescent multiple myeloma cells. Blood. 2014;123(14):2204–8.
72. Lawson MA, McDonald MM, Kovacic N, Hua Khoo W, Terry RL, Down J, et al. Osteoclasts control reactivation of dormant myeloma cells by remodelling the endosteal niche. Nat Commun. 2015;6:8983.
73. Berenson JR, Lichtenstein A, Porter L, Dimopoulos MA, Bordoni R, George S, et al. Efficacy of pamidronate in reducing skeletal events in patients with advanced multiple myeloma. Myeloma Aredia Study Group. N Engl J Med. 1996;334(8):488–93.
74. Rosen LS, Gordon D, Kaminski M, Howell A, Belch A, Mackey J, et al. Zoledronic acid versus pamidronate in the treatment of skeletal metastases in patients with breast cancer or osteolytic lesions of multiple myeloma: a phase III, double-blind, comparative trial. Cancer J. 2001;7(5):377–87.
75. Gimsing P, Carlson K, Turesson I, Fayers P, Waage A, Vangsted A, et al. Effect of pamidronate 30 mg versus 90 mg on physical

function in patients with newly diagnosed multiple myeloma (Nordic Myeloma Study Group): a double-blind, randomised controlled trial. Lancet Oncol. 2010;11(10):973–82.
76. Morgan GJ, Davies FE, Gregory WM, Cocks K, Bell SE, Szubert AJ, et al. First-line treatment with zoledronic acid as compared with clodronic acid in multiple myeloma (MRC Myeloma IX): a randomised controlled trial. Lancet. 2010;376(9757):1989–99.
77. Morgan GJ, Child JA, Gregory WM, Szubert AJ, Cocks K, Bell SE, et al. Effects of zoledronic acid versus clodronic acid on skeletal morbidity in patients with newly diagnosed multiple myeloma (MRC Myeloma IX): secondary outcomes from a randomised controlled trial. Lancet Oncol. 2011;12(8):743–52.
78. Himelstein AL, Foster JC, Khatcheressian JL, Roberts JD, Seisler DK, Novotny PJ, et al. Effect of longer-interval vs standard dosing of zoledronic acid on skeletal events in patients with bone metastases: a randomized clinical trial. JAMA. 2017;317(1):48–58.
79. van Beek E, Pieterman E, Cohen L, Lowik C, Papapoulos S. Farnesyl pyrophosphate synthase is the molecular target of nitrogen-containing bisphosphonates. Biochem Biophys Res Commun. 1999;264(1):108–11.
80. Croucher PI, De Hendrik R, Perry MJ, Hijzen A, Shipman CM, Lippitt J, et al. Zoledronic acid treatment of 5T2MM-bearing mice inhibits the development of myeloma bone disease: evidence for decreased osteolysis, tumor burden and angiogenesis, and increased survival. J Bone Miner Res. 2003;18(3):482–92.
81. Mhaskar R, Kumar A, Miladinovic B, Djulbegovic B. Bisphosphonates in multiple myeloma: an updated network meta-analysis. Cochrane Database Syst Rev. 2017;12:CD003188.
82. Guenther A, Gordon S, Tiemann M, Burger R, Bakker F, Green JR, et al. The bisphosphonate zoledronic acid has antimyeloma activity in vivo by inhibition of protein prenylation. Int J Cancer. 2010;126(1):239–46.
83. Corso A, Ferretti E, Lunghi M, Zappasodi P, Mangiacavalli S, De Amici M, et al. Zoledronic acid down-regulates adhesion molecules of bone marrow stromal cells in multiple myeloma: a possible mechanism for its antitumor effect. Cancer. 2005;104(1):118–25.
84. Terpos E, Kleber M, Engelhardt M, Zweegman S, Gay F, Kastritis E, et al. European Myeloma Network guidelines for the management of multiple myeloma-related complications. Haematologica. 2015;100(10):1254–66.

85. Kanellias N, Gavriatopoulou M, Terpos E, Dimopoulos MA. Management of multiple myeloma bone disease: impact of treatment on renal function. Expert Rev Hematol. 2018;11(11):881–8.
86. Kyle RA, Yee GC, Somerfield MR, Flynn PJ, Halabi S, Jagannath S, et al. American Society of Clinical Oncology 2007 clinical practice guideline update on the role of bisphosphonates in multiple myeloma. J Clin Oncol. 2007;25(17):2464–72.
87. Black DM, Kelly MP, Genant HK, Palermo L, Eastell R, Bucci-Rechtweg C, et al. Bisphosphonates and fractures of the subtrochanteric or diaphyseal femur. N Engl J Med. 2010;362(19):1761–71.
88. Herrera L, Leal I, Lapi F, Schuemie M, Arcoraci V, Cipriani F, et al. Risk of atrial fibrillation among bisphosphonate users: a multicenter, population-based, Italian study. Osteoporos Int. 2015;26(5):1499–506.
89. Wang JC, Chien WC, Chung CH, Liao WI, Tsai SH. Adverse cardiovascular effects of nitrogen-containing bisphosphonates in patients with osteoporosis: a nationwide population-based retrospective study. Int J Cardiol. 2016;215:232–7.
90. Terpos E, Morgan G, Dimopoulos MA, Drake MT, Lentzsch S, Raje N, et al. International Myeloma Working Group recommendations for the treatment of multiple myeloma-related bone disease. J Clin Oncol. 2013;31(18):2347–57.
91. Body JJ, Facon T, Coleman RE, Lipton A, Geurs F, Fan M, et al. A study of the biological receptor activator of nuclear factor-kappaB ligand inhibitor, denosumab, in patients with multiple myeloma or bone metastases from breast cancer. Clin Cancer Res. 2006;12(4):1221–8.
92. Kostenuik PJ, Nguyen HQ, McCabe J, Warmington KS, Kurahara C, Sun N, et al. Denosumab, a fully human monoclonal antibody to RANKL, inhibits bone resorption and increases BMD in knock-in mice that express chimeric (murine/human) RANKL. J Bone Miner Res. 2009;24(2):182–95.
93. Vij R, Horvath N, Spencer A, Taylor K, Vadhan-Raj S, Vescio R, et al. An open-label, phase 2 trial of denosumab in the treatment of relapsed or plateau-phase multiple myeloma. Am J Hematol. 2009;84(10):650–6.
94. Fizazi K, Bosserman L, Gao G, Skacel T, Markus R. Denosumab treatment of prostate cancer with bone metastases and increased urine N-telopeptide levels after therapy with intrave-

nous bisphosphonates: results of a randomized phase II trial. J Urol. 2009;182(2):509–15; discussion 15–6
95. Terpos E, Willenbacher W, Shimizu K, García-Sanz R, Glennane A, Guan X, et al. Progression-free survival subset analysis – denosumab vs zoledronic acid in bone disease treatment of newly diagnosed multiple myeloma: an international, double-blind, double-dummy, randomized controlled phase 3 study. Blood. 2018;132:1969.
96. Terpos E, Ntanasis-Stathopoulos I, Dimopoulos MA. Myeloma bone disease: from biology findings to treatment approaches. Blood. 2019;133(14):1534–9.
97. Tsourdi E, Langdahl B, Cohen-Solal M, Aubry-Rozier B, Eriksen EF, Guanabens N, et al. Discontinuation of Denosumab therapy for osteoporosis: a systematic review and position statement by ECTS. Bone. 2017;105:11–7.
98. Leder BZ, Tsai JN, Jiang LA, Lee H. Importance of prompt antiresorptive therapy in postmenopausal women discontinuing teriparatide or denosumab: The Denosumab and Teriparatide Follow-up study (DATA-Follow-up). Bone. 2017;98:54–8.
99. Block GA, Bone HG, Fang L, Lee E, Padhi D. A single-dose study of denosumab in patients with various degrees of renal impairment. J Bone Miner Res. 2012;27(7):1471–9.
100. Stopeck AT, Lipton A, Body JJ, Steger GG, Tonkin K, de Boer RH, et al. Denosumab compared with zoledronic acid for the treatment of bone metastases in patients with advanced breast cancer: a randomized, double-blind study. J Clin Oncol. 2010;28(35):5132–9.
101. Saad F, Brown JE, Van Poznak C, Ibrahim T, Stemmer SM, Stopeck AT, et al. Incidence, risk factors, and outcomes of osteonecrosis of the jaw: integrated analysis from three blinded active-controlled phase III trials in cancer patients with bone metastases. Ann Oncol. 2012;23(5):1341–7.
102. Woo SB, Hellstein JW, Kalmar JR. Narrative [corrected] review: bisphosphonates and osteonecrosis of the jaws. Ann Intern Med. 2006;144(10):753–61.
103. Cosman F, Crittenden DB, Adachi JD, Binkley N, Czerwinski E, Ferrari S, et al. Romosozumab treatment in postmenopausal women with osteoporosis. N Engl J Med. 2016;375(16):1532–43.
104. McClung MR, Grauer A, Boonen S, Bolognese MA, Brown JP, Diez-Perez A, et al. Romosozumab in postmenopausal women with low bone mineral density. N Engl J Med. 2014;370(5):412–20.

105. Padhi D, Jang G, Stouch B, Fang L, Posvar E. Single-dose, placebo-controlled, randomized study of AMG 785, a sclerostin monoclonal antibody. J Bone Miner Res. 2011;26(1):19–26.
106. Graeff C, Campbell GM, Pena J, Borggrefe J, Padhi D, Kaufman A, et al. Administration of romosozumab improves vertebral trabecular and cortical bone as assessed with quantitative computed tomography and finite element analysis. Bone. 2015;81:364–9.
107. Raje N, Roodman GD, Willenbacher W, Shimizu K, Garcia-Sanz R, Terpos E, et al. A cost-effectiveness analysis of denosumab for the prevention of skeletal-related events in patients with multiple myeloma in the United States of America. J Med Econ. 2018;21(5):525–36

Chapter 8
Orthopaedic Management in Multiple Myeloma: What Is the Role and When?

Karen L. Shepherd and Gillian L. Cribb

Introduction

Involvement of the orthopaedic surgeon with patients and myeloma is multifaceted; Investigation and diagnosis of one or more bone lesions as the first manifestation of malignancy, or a skeletal-related event (SRE) with a known history of myeloma. Orthopaedic surgeons commonly diagnose myeloma and manage the bone sequelae of the disease particularly in the spine and long bones.

Skeletal-related events include bone pain, fracture and cord compression or compromise. In the myeloma population,

K. L. Shepherd (✉) · G. L. Cribb
Montgomery Unit, The Robert Jones and Agnes Hunt Orthopaedic Hospital NHS Foundation Trust, Oswestry, UK
e-mail: karen.shepherd15@nhs.net

E. Zamagni (ed.), *Management of Bone Disease and Kidney Failure in Multiple Myeloma*,
https://doi.org/10.1007/978-3-030-63662-3_8

the incidence of SREs is over 34% [1]. Referrals for patients presenting in this manner are made via general practitioners, the emergency department and from generalist orthopaedic surgeons to subsite or super specialist orthopaedic services such as orthopaedic oncology or spinal surgeons. This is often a result of noted abnormal imaging performed to investigate bone pain or presentation with fracture or neurological change. Communication pathways between other specialties including haematology and oncology (particularly cancer of unknown primary – CUP teams) are crucial. Diagnosis may require a targeted bone biopsy, usually when metastatic carcinoma has been excluded or the myeloma lesion is non-secretory. Continued communication between haematology and orthopaedics is also essential in the long-term management of patients with bone lesions at risk of pathological fracture.

Presentation

Bone pain in myeloma presents when the integrity of the bone is compromised in its normal function – such as pain on weight-bearing if the tumour disrupts the periosteum or the tumour volume causes pressure effects on surrounding structures. Given myeloma is a marrow disease, periosteal disruption is a late sign. It is therefore more likely to cause structural weakness only after it has invaded the stronger cortical bone. Lesions are also commonly found in locations where the pressure effects can hide for some time, such as the pelvis. Pain reported from these areas is usually vague, with physical functioning of the affected area declining slowly over time. When the lesion compresses the nerves, the presentation may mimic radiculopathy. In spinal disease patients can present as per the spectrum of metastatic cord compression or in the fracture clinic as vertebral collapse, mimicking osteoporotic signs and symptoms.

Case Examples of Presenting Features

Pathological Fracture Leading to New Diagnosis

It is relatively rare for patients to present to the orthopaedic surgeon as a new diagnosis, with fracture as a result of myeloma. The most common scenario is the elderly patient, with chronic hip pain attributed to degenerative change, admitted with a pathological fracture of the proximal femur (fractured hip). When a new patient with a pathological fracture is identified, the diagnostic process should be followed as per guidelines. This is detailed further in the chapter.

Pain and Abnormal X-Ray, with Normal Myeloma Screen

Radiograph is slightly abnormal but inconclusive; plasma electrophoresis and urine Bence Jones protein are negative. No history of malignancy. This is extremely challenging to the general practitioner. Some regions will have a musculoskeletal tumour service and are ideally placed to investigate this. Other patients may be referred into the local CUP team. Patients are likely to undergo further imaging including CT chest, abdomen and pelvis (Figs. 8.1 and 8.2) and whole body nuclear medicine bone scan. No primary identified. This patient will require further imaging of the bone, including MRI, and a biopsy of the lesion. Non-secretory myeloma is a challenge to diagnose, and a targeted bone biopsy is often necessary.

Summary of the Principles of Management

1. Confirm diagnosis by either haematological investigations or bone biopsy
2. Indications for bone biopsy

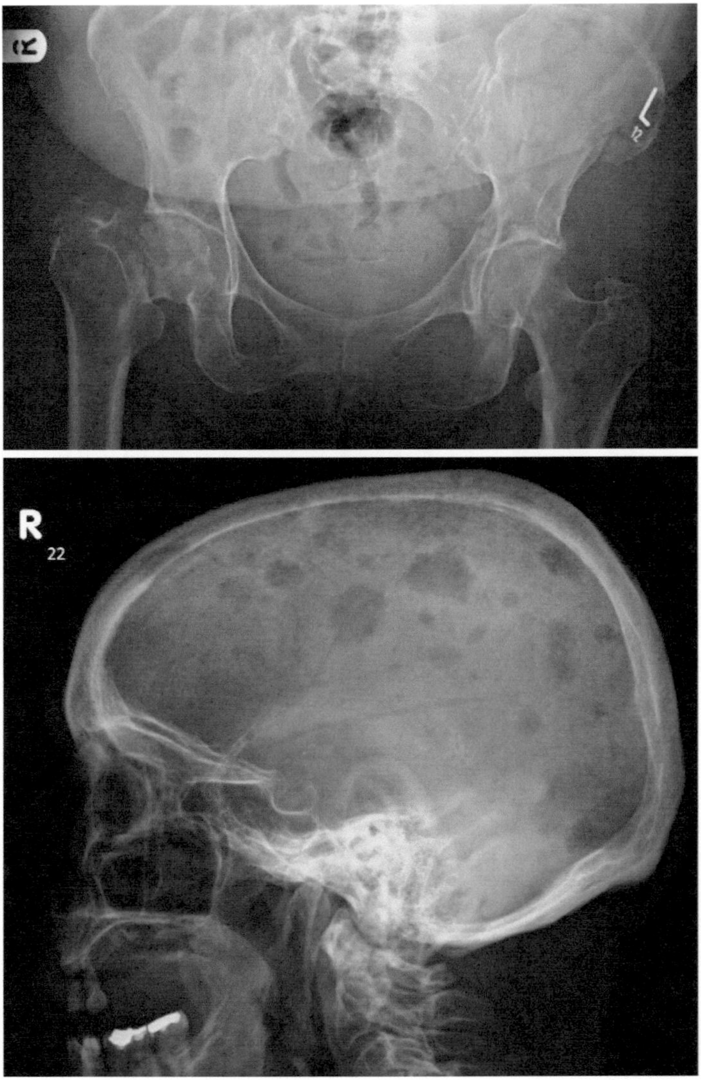

FIGURE 8.1 Presented with 2-week history of groin pain. Further imaging suggestive of myeloma

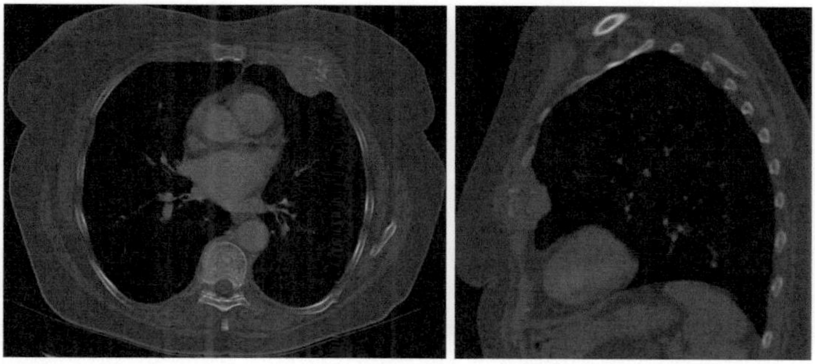

FIGURE 8.2 Presented as an isolated bone lesion in the rib. Managed as per a primary bone tumour. Plasma cell tumour on biopsy

- Negative haematological investigations
- Long disease-free interval
- Imaging and presentation are atypical – consider new metastatic non-myelomatous disease or primary bone tumour if solitary.

3. The British Orthopaedic Oncology Society (BOOS) and British Orthopaedic Association (BOA) metastatic bone disease guidelines [2] are an excellent basis to consider a best practice approach to orthopaedic manifestations of haematological bone disease. The diagnostic and outcome principles are largely similar. Nuances exist with regard surgical management. Pertinent summary points from the guidelines are as follows:

- Any interventional treatment must improve quality of life
- Implant choice should last the life time of the patient
- Consider symptoms and fracture risk (related to location)
- Consider prognosis
- Stage disease and consider physiological reserve
- Liaison with haematology

Staging and Confirmation of Diagnosis via Bone Biopsy

Any patient with a suspicious solitary bone lesion should be investigated with a full clinical history and examination, followed by investigation with routine blood tests (FBC, U&E, LFT, bone profile, ESR, CRP and tumour markers) and radiological investigations (Fig. 8.3). Whole body nuclear medicine bone scan for myeloma can be challenging to interpret in the presence of fracture (hot), when myeloma overall can display minimal uptake. The case should then be

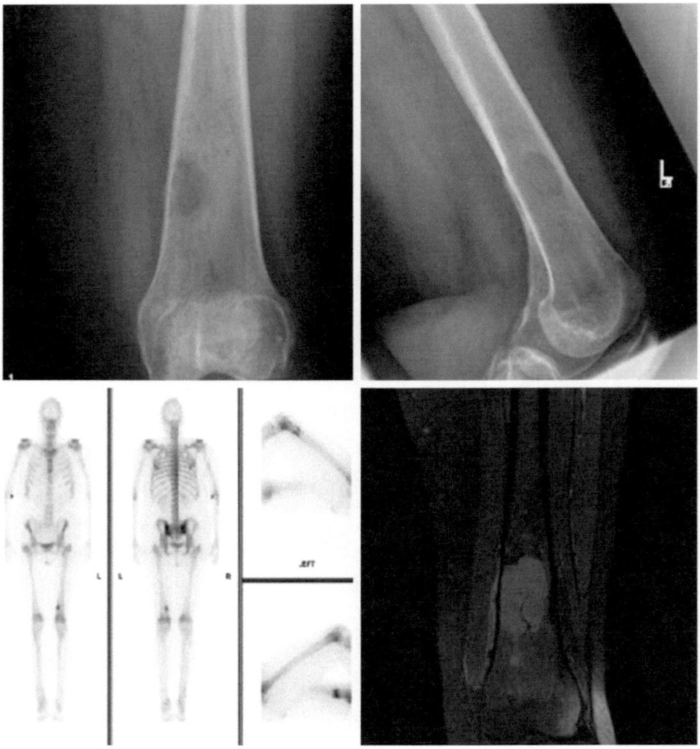

FIGURE 8.3 Full staging (including a CT chest, abdomen and pelvis) for bone tumour investigation

discussed in a multidisciplinary team (MDT) setting, including surgeon and radiologist input for planning image-guided percutaneous biopsy.

Metastatic or haematological malignant bone disease is managed initially via a similar route. Diagnosis confirmation is a priority. The indications for bone biopsy include negative or inconclusive myeloma screen (blood and urine tests) and no primary tumour identified on imaging. In patients who have a previous known malignancy with a long disease-free interval or the bone disease is atypical, a biopsy is also indicated. Bone biopsy may be performed if accessibility to biopsy of other lesions is challenging.

Each centre should have a detailed protocol and system for biopsy (Figs. 8.4 and 8.5). The biopsy should be performed in a centre that has the appropriate skills and personnel to optimise the true positive biopsy rate. This involves appro-

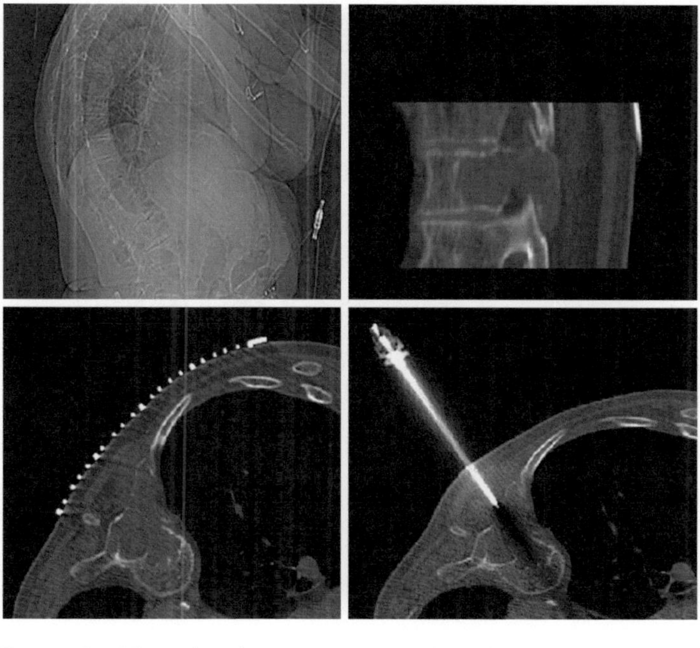

FIGURE 8.4 Thoracic spine percutaneous CT-guided biopsy

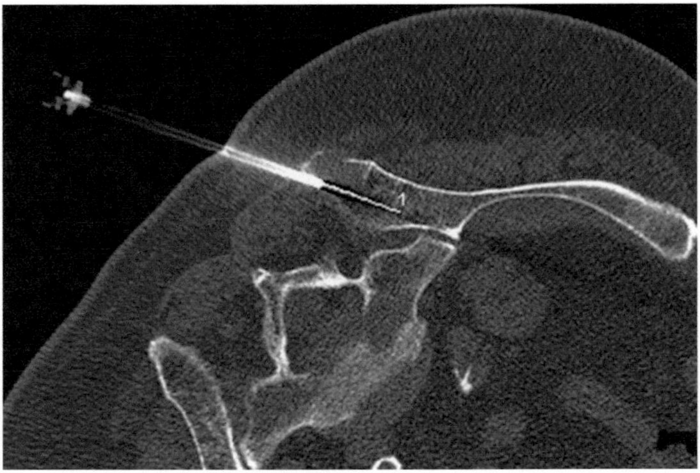

FIGURE 8.5 Posterior ilium percutaneous CT-guided biopsy

priate clinical review, MDT assessment and radiological and pathological expertise. Bone biopsy is painful. Consideration should be given to adequate analgesia to minimise patient distress and reduce movement artefact. General or regional anaesthesia are recommended options, especially for deeper and anatomically sensitive locations.

Decision-Making

Any management decision for a patient with myeloma and SRE should be considered to undergo MDT review – both haematological and surgical. The direction of any decision is also influenced by whether the patient is newly diagnosed with myeloma, has refractory disease or has limited therapeutic options in either the haematological or orthopaedic specialties. It is expected that newly diagnosed patients have more oncological options, and therefore surgery could be delayed or indeed averted.

From a surgical perspective the considerations are;

- Nature of the symptoms and their magnitude/impact
  - Quality of life for the patient living with the disease and symptoms
- Fracture risk
  - The risks for prophylactic management compared to treatment following fracture
- Potential for improvement with medical/oncological management and interim risks for bone stability and/or malignant spinal cord compression
- Fitness for surgery
  - Comorbid status

    Biological age, performance status, patient motivation and compliance
  - Prognosis
  - Disease progression and status regarding oncological input (e.g. whether the patient has exhausted all medical options)
  - Review medications. Targeted therapies and anticoagulation may require cessation/delay. It should be questioned as to how this will affect systemic disease

The aims of any management plan for patients with malignant bone disease are to maintain their function and independence and minimise pain. Surgery has a clear negative impact in the short term. The decision-making therefore is crucial to the medium- and long-term outcomes for these patients.

Orthopaedic Management Options

Nonoperative

The majority of patients with myeloma will not require the services of an orthopaedic surgeon. Oncological therapies including chemotherapy, targeted therapies and radiotherapy are the mainstay of medical management. Bone-specific targeting drugs including bisphosphonates and denosumab also have an important role. Unless the patient requires emergent orthopaedic input, for pathological fracture, imminent fracture, intractable pain or spinal compromise, patients should be managed by the haematologist. It is recommended that patients continue to be followed up in the orthopaedic setting if there is a potential requirement for surgery in the future (Fig. 8.6).

Operative

The role of the orthopaedic surgeon is to treat the myelomatous deposits for pain and to prevent fracture, to stabilise or reconstruct pathological fracture and to decompress the spinal cord/nerve roots and stabilise spinal instability. In disease affecting the appendicular skeleton, the most critical are load-bearing long bones such as the femur, tibia and humerus. Orthopaedic management must be patient specific, individualised and both haematological and patient opinions considered. In addition to multiple myeloma as a diagnosis, we must also consider the role of surgery in rare isolated disease – plasmacytoma. This requires discussion between haematologists and the surgeon. Arguably the management and thus the indications for surgery should be the same as for multiple myeloma.

Where the management of haematological bone disease can differ from that of metastatic bone disease the decision is between stabilisation and excision. Stabilisation involves internal fixation techniques such as plates and screws and

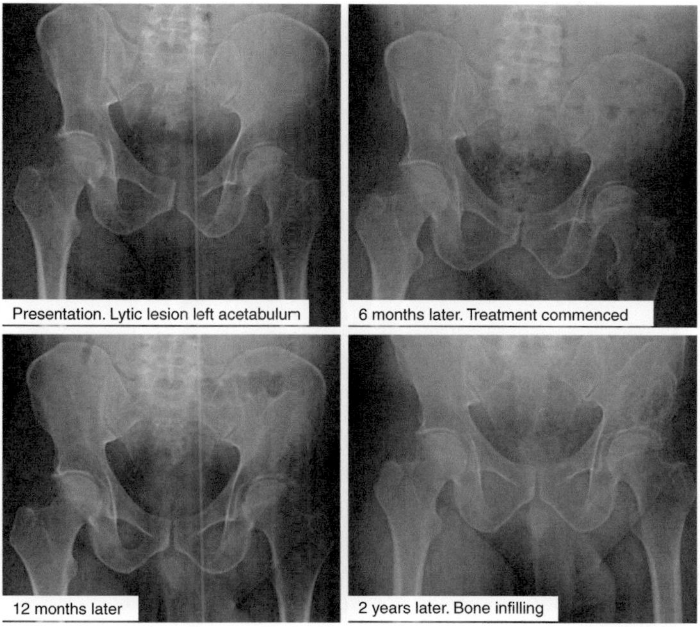

FIGURE 8.6 Patient presented with groin pain. Lesion left superior acetabulum. Myeloma. No surgery. Treated with bortezomib, thalidomide and dexamethasone, zoledronic acid and stem cell transplant

intramedullary devices ('nail' or 'pin'). Excision involves the removal of the malignant area of the bone, with reconstruction using arthroplasty implants such as a hip or knee replacement. Haematological malignancies are considered more radiosensitive and are known to have an increased healing capacity than solid organ metastases. Therefore, internal fixation methods may have a stronger role in these patients, especially if external beam radiotherapy can be given post-operatively.

Minimum standards of care must include evaluation of potential for fracture union and disease progression and consideration to impending or failure of reconstruction. The implant should last the lifetime of the patient. Fixation methods will fail if the tumour does not response to therapy. Excision should be considered over internal fixation (Fig. 8.7)

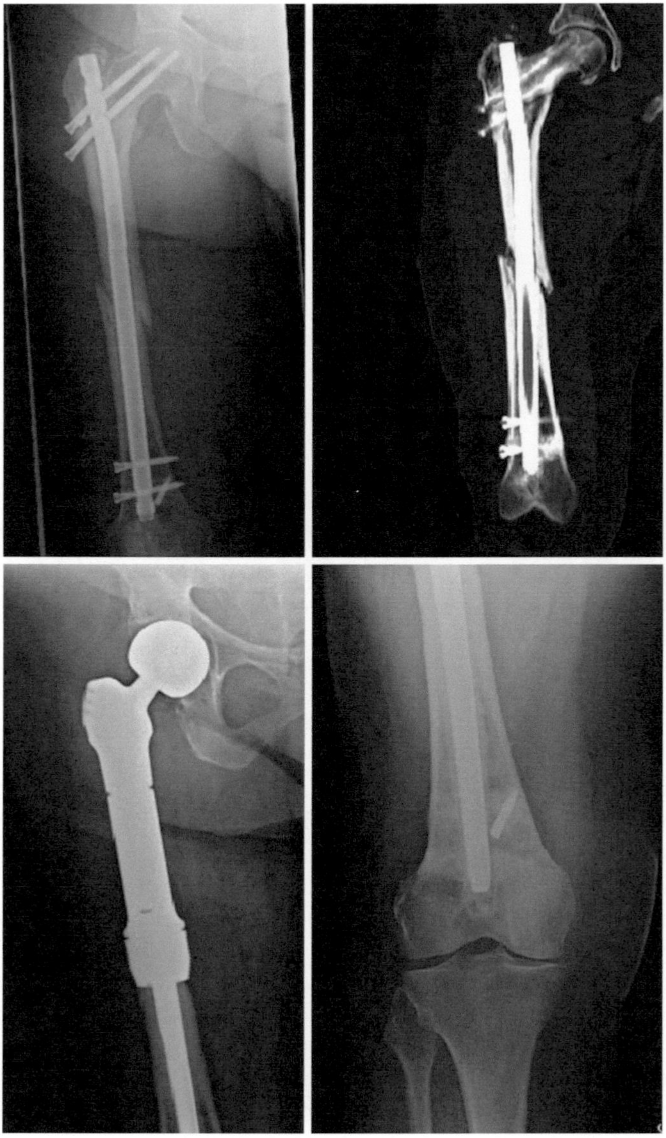

FIGURE 8.7 Mid-shaft pathological fracture. Intramedullary nail inserted. Non-union with broken metalwork (proximal and distal screws). Revision surgery to excision with endoprosthetic replacement reconstruction 3 years later

if concern exists as to the potential for bone healing (previous radiotherapy, end-stage disease, anatomical location). Mechanical pain is not managed merely by internal fixation, bone healing is required. Orthopaedic follow up is required post-operatively to monitor healing and/or fixation failure.

Types of Implants and Reconstruction

Internal Fixation (Figs. 8.8, 8.9, 8.10 and 8.11)

Resection and Replacement Surgery (Figs. 8.12 and 8.13)

Risks

The risks of surgical intervention for patients with myeloma can be categorised as perioperative or late.

Preoperatively an assessment of physiologic reserve and therefore the ability to cope with the trauma of the surgical insult is essential. The blood indices and their trend are known valuable indicators in metastatic disease and myeloma [3, 4]. Patients should undergo anaesthetic-led preoperative assessment, where the trends of blood tests and specifically haemoglobin, clotting, albumin and renal function are evaluated. The main risks discussed within the consent process are infection, bleeding, thromboembolic disease, cardiovascular events and death. Myelomatous lesions have the potential for significant blood loss, and perioperative planning is key to safety.

Later risks or concerns are non-union (non-healing of the bone), ongoing pain, symptomatic metalwork, metalwork failure and loss of function.

Given the potential to decrease a patients' quality of life and indeed shorten the life expectancy, consent should follow the clear principles of consent outlined by the GMC [5].

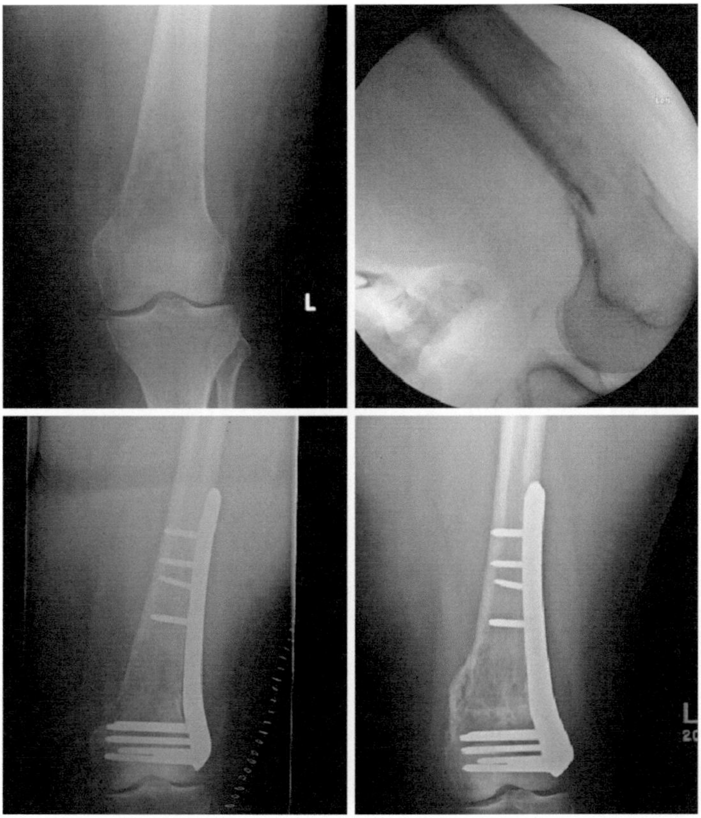

Figure 8.8 Referred with pathological fracture left distal femur. Biopy, followed by internal fixation (plate and screws). Oncological management: bortezomib, cyclophosphamide, dexamethasone and zoledronic acid post-operatively together with radiotherapy. Post-op images 1 year later

In summary, optimised patients with myeloma, who undergo surgery that has been appropriately considered, usually have favourable outcomes given the sensitivity of the disease to medical therapies. Surgery is an adjunct to these therapies. Communication between the haematology and orthopaedic oncology MDT groups is fundamental to outcomes.

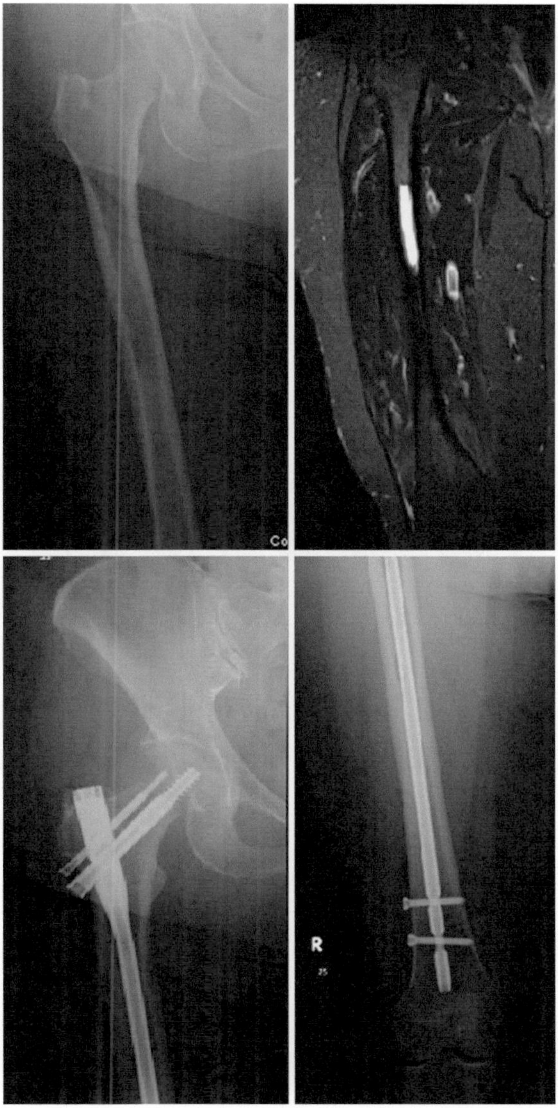

FIGURE 8.9 Right femoral diaphysis lesion. Monitored for 6 months (initially asymptomatic). Pain and difficulty weight-bearing (MRI performed) and endosteal erosion noted on CT. Intramedullary nail inserted followed by radiotherapy. No progression of lesion

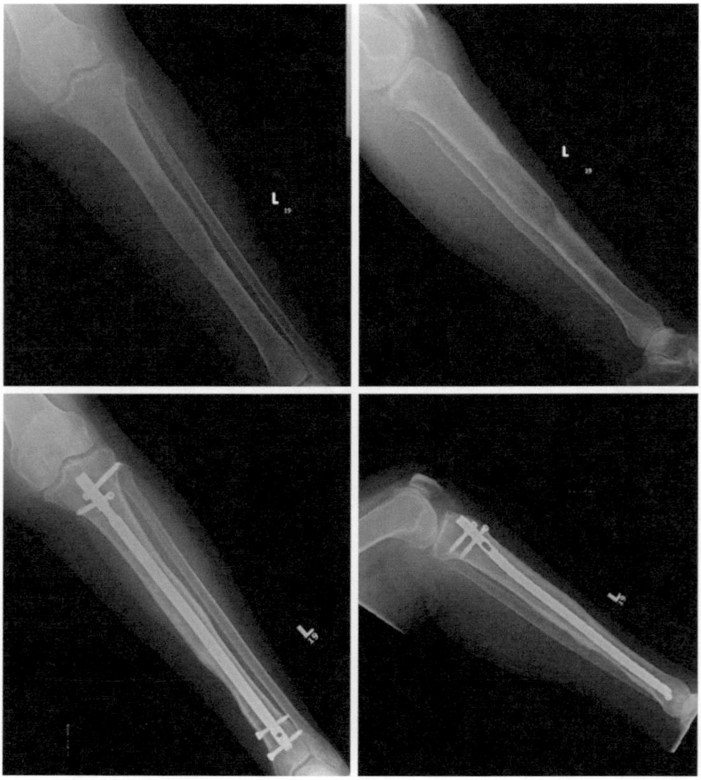

Figure 8.10 Left tibia intramedullary nail. Increasing symptoms from a diaphyseal lesion over 3 years. End-stage oncological treatment. Surgery followed by radiotherapy with resolution of symptoms. Local recurrence 1 year later and died 18 months following surgery with minimal symptoms in the leg

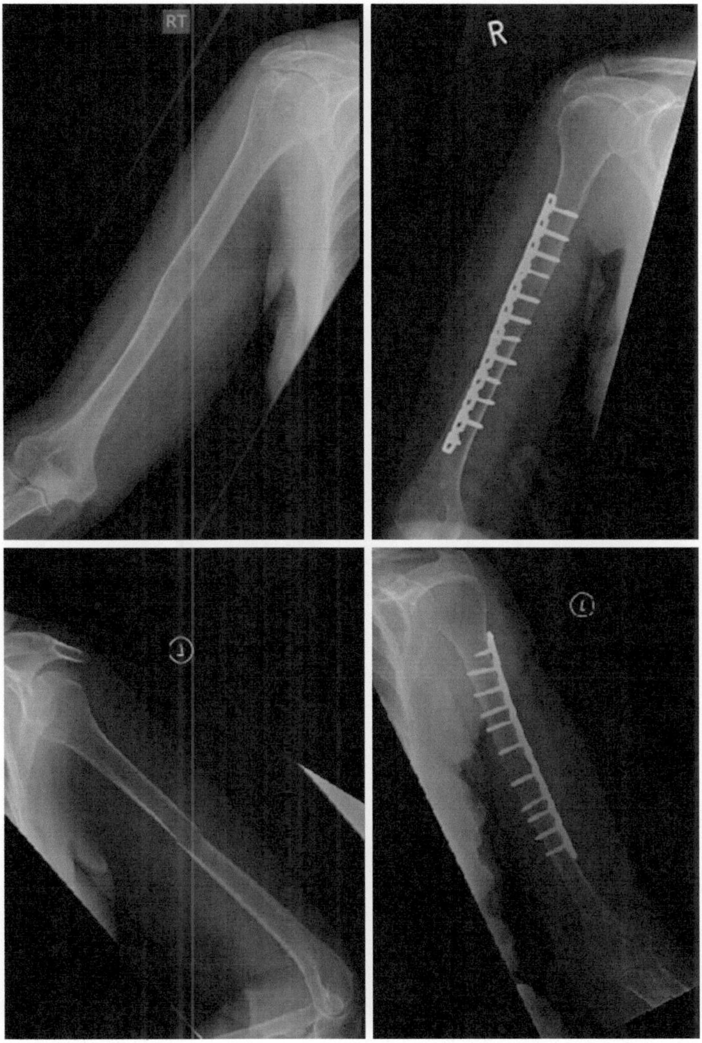

FIGURE 8.11 Bilateral humeri lesions. Both underwent internal fixation followed by radiotherapy

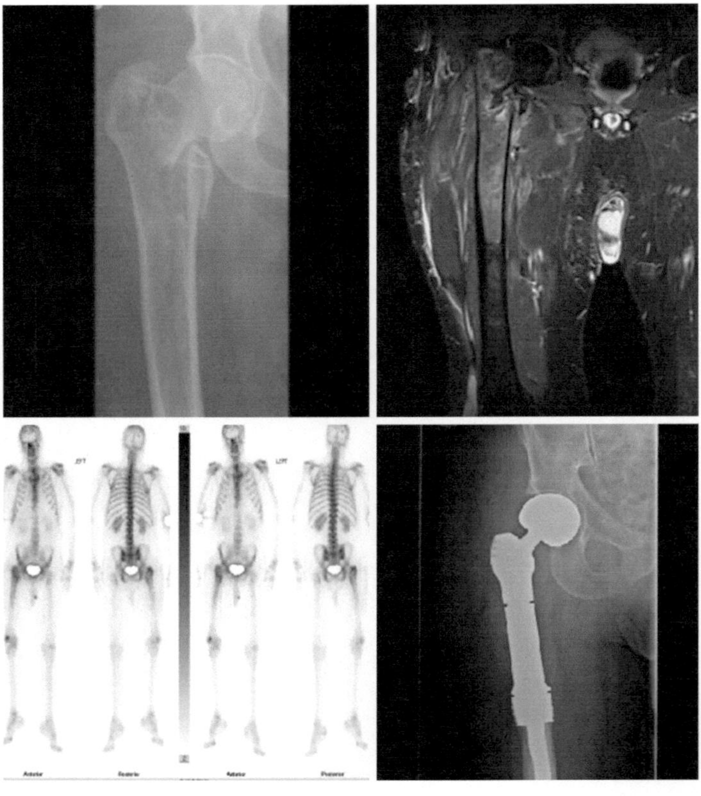

FIGURE 8.12 Right proximal femoral lesion. First presentation. Given extensive cortical compromise, endoprosthetic replacement performed. Referred to haematology post-operatively

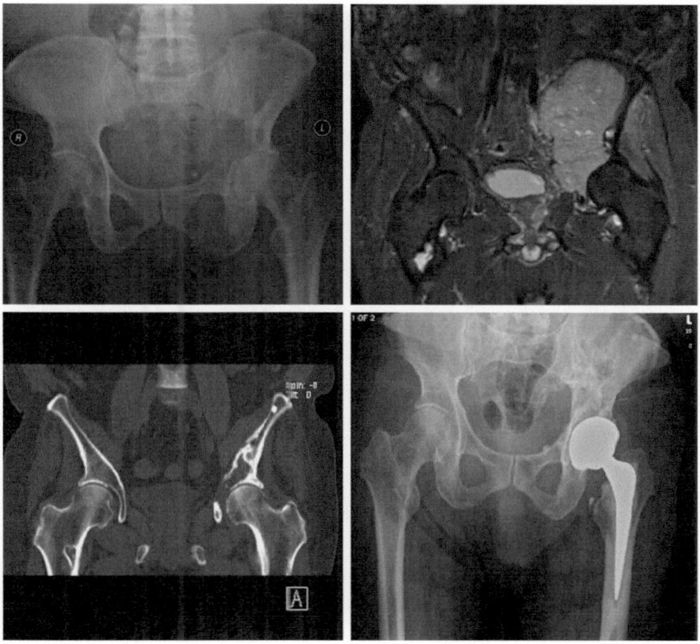

FIGURE 8.13 Left acetabular myeloma with pathological fracture. Following chemotherapy, the bone consolidated, and this was reconstructed with a standard total hip replacement. The lesion was unreconstructable prior to bone consolidation

References

1. Kim C, Bhatta S, Cyprien L, Fonseca R, Hernandez RK. Incidence of skeletal-related events among multiple myeloma patients in the United States at oncology clinics: observations from real-world data. J Bone Oncol. 2018;14:100215. https://doi.org/10.1016/j.jbo.2018.100215. PMID: 30666288; PMCID: PMC6329702.
2. Tillman RM, Ashford RU. Metastatic bone disease: a guide to good practice. 2013 Revision. British Orthopaedic Association. https://www.boa.ac.uk/wp-content/uploads/2014/01/Metastatic-Bone-Disease.pdf. Accessed 01/01/2020.
3. Shepherd KL. Controversies in the management of metastatic bones disease. J Trauma Orthopaed Surg. 2017;6(4):58–60.

4. Greipp PR, Miguel JS, Durie BGM, Crowley JJ, Barlogie B, Bladé J, Boccadoro M, Child JA, Avet-Loiseau H, Harousseau J-L, Kyle RA, Lahuerta JJ, Ludwig H, Morgan G, Powles R, Shimizu K, Shustik C, Sonneveld P, Tosi P, IngemarTuresson JW. International staging system for multiple myeloma. J Clin Oncol. 2005;23(15):3412–20.
5. Consent: patients and doctors making decisions together. The General Medical Council. https://www.gmc-uk.org/ethical-guidance/ethical-guidance-for-doctors/consent. Accessed 01/01/2020.

Chapter 9
The Pathophysiology of Kidney Involvement in Multiple Myeloma and Monoclonal-Related Disorders

Valeria Corradetti, Giorgia Comai, Claudia Bini, and Gaetano La Manna

Epidemiology of Renal Injury in Multiple Myeloma (MM) and Monoclonal-Related Disorders

Multiple myeloma is the most common malignancy associated with end-stage renal disease (ESRD), and 20–50% of patients have renal involvement at diagnosis, presenting as end-stage renal disease approximately in 1% of cases [1–3]. The European and US registries demonstrate that 1.8–4.5% of the ESRD population is affected by multiple myeloma, and patients are prevalently men older than 65 years old [1, 4].

V. Corradetti · G. Comai · C. Bini · G. La Manna (✉)
Department of Experimental Diagnostic and Specialty Medicine (DIMES), Nephrology, Dialysis and Renal Transplant Unit, S. Orsola-Malpighi Hospital, University of Bologna, Bologna, Italy
e-mail: Giorgia.comai@aosp.bo.it; gaetano.lamanna@unibo.it

E. Zamagni (ed.), *Management of Bone Disease and Kidney Failure in Multiple Myeloma*,
https://doi.org/10.1007/978-3-030-63662-3_9

Moreover, renal involvement in MM has a documented importance in prognosis. In fact, the median survival of patients with MM is reduced when renal involvement is present, although the new therapeutic approaches have improved prognosis [5]. Moreover, there is growing evidence that a prompt reduction of free light chains (FLC) from circulation both by chemotherapy and plasmapheresis can lead to renal recovery and there is a percentage of patients escaping dialysis [1, 6–12].

Recently, it has been recognized a small number of patients, about 1.5%, with a monoclonal gammopathy of undetermined significance (MGUS) that present renaldysfunction and pathological findings on renal biopsy related to monoclonal immunoglobulin [13–15]. This disease entity has been defined in 2012 with the term "monoclonal gammopathy of renal significance" (MGRS) that describes all B cell or plasma cell proliferative disorders that produce a monoclonal immunoglobulin associated with kidney injury [15]. These diseases tend to be progressive and are unlikely to undergo spontaneous remission or to respond to conventional immunosuppression; clone-directed therapies are required to prevent further kidney damage resulting in end-stage renal disease [13, 16–23].

Clinical Presentation

The clinical features of renal involvement in immunoglobulin-related disorders are heterogeneous and often reflect a different pathological pattern. The presence of renal involvement is one of the essential criteria for multiple myeloma definition, specifically the presence of renal impairment and a serum creatinine >2.0 mg/dl related to the plasma cell dyscrasia [24]. The clinical presentation pattern is variable and depends on the histological damage, as shown in Fig. 9.1 [25, 26].

Renal involvement can present acutely in the form of acute kidney injury (AKI), in 1–5% of cases requiring dia-

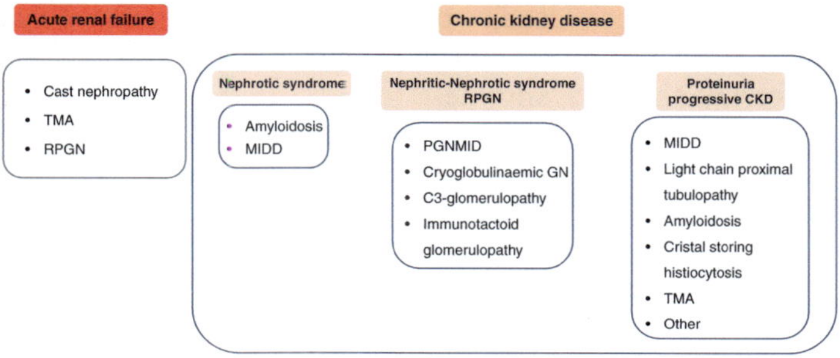

FIGURE 9.1 Typical clinical features of renal injury associated with monoclonal immunoglobulin. Ig immunoglobulin, TMA thrombotic microangiopathy, CKD chronic kidney disease, MIDD monoclonal immunoglobulin deposition disease, RPGN rapidly progressive glomerulonephritis, PGNMID proliferative glomerulonephritis with monoclonal Ig deposits

lytic treatment. Recovery of renal function occurs in less than 25% of patients who require dialysis [1, 4]. In these cases the most frequent histological feature is cast nephropathy that represents about 40% of the histological patterns at renal biopsy.

An extremely rare presentation of renal involvement in the form of AKI is thrombotic microangiopathy. It represented only the 0.5% of renal lesions in a cohort of 190 patients with multiple myeloma, although when it associates to monoclonal Ig-related disorders, the evolution of renal involvement in ESRD is 50% compared to the 33% probability of patients without thrombotic microangiopathy [25, 26]. The clinical manifestation is characterized by signs of intravascular hemolysis, acute kidney injury, microhematuria, and a non-nephrotic proteinuria.

Renal involvement in monoclonal Ig-related disorders can manifest in the form of slow, progressive renal damage associated with different grades of proteinuria, hematuria, or Fanconi syndrome.

AL amyloidosis usually presents with different grade of renal dysfunction associated with nephrotic range proteinuria or overt nephrotic syndrome.

When the glomerulus is directly involved, the clinical presentation may be as a rapidly progressive decline in renal function (RPGN, rapidly progressive glomerulonephritis) or a chronic dysfunction associated with nephritic proteinuria or nephrotic syndrome; this is the case of proliferative glomerulonephritis, C3 glomerulopathy, immunotactoid glomerulonephritis, or monoclonal immunoglobulin deposition in the glomerulus.

Another possible presentation is chronic kidney dysfunction associated with Fanconi syndrome; this clinical picture reflects histological involvement of the tubules, as in light chain proximal tubulopathy or monoclonal immunoglobulin deposition disease.

Immunoglobulins and Free Light Chain Physiology

The proliferating clone in plasma cell dyscrasias is associated with the production of monoclonal immunoglobulin (Ig) and of a variable quantity of free light chains (FLC).

In healthy conditions Ig heavy chains cannot be filtered by the glomerulus due to their large dimensions (molecular weight >60 kDa) and are removed from circulation by pinocytosis (IgA and IgG) or by pinocytosis and recycling by FcRn receptors (IgM) [27–30].

FLC production is about 40% more than Ig, and about 500 mg/day are released in circulation; the 80% is distributed in the extravascular space [31–33]. Two-thirds of light chain production are of κ type, resulting in a serum κ/λ ratio of 1.8:1 [34]. FLC κ are monomers of a molecular weight of around 25 kDa and have a renal clearance of 40% per hour, with a serum half-life of 2–4 hours. FLC λ circulate as dimers of around 50 kDa and have a renal clearance of 20% per hour with a serum half-life of 3–6 hours [32, 35–38]. When the renal clearance reduces, as in chronic kidney disease, κ and λ FLC concentrations increase and a greater proportion of FLC is removed through pinocytosis by cells of the reticuloendothelial system [36, 39].

The kidneys filter about 0.5–1 g/day of FLC, after filtration FLC are bound by megalin and cubilin receptors on brush border of the proximal tubule epithelium with a fast and saturable endocytotic process. There they are completely adsorbed and hydrolyzed by lysozymes and the resulting amino acids return to the circulation. The urinary excretion of FLC is unremarkable, about 1–10 mg/day, originating by secretion processes [40–45].

FLC Metabolism and Mechanisms of Injury During Monoclonal Clone-Related Disorders

During plasma cell dyscrasias, the production of FLC increases and is predominantly monoclonal, and circulating FLC amounts can rise to levels as high as 100 g/L. In fact, the kidneys may filter over 80 g/day of FLC. As a consequence, proximal tubular reabsorption is saturated and FLC are excreted in the urine, known as Bence Jones proteinuria [46, 47]. In contrast, circulating Ig is not filtered by the glomerulus.

Since the 1990s, it is known that FLC isolated from patients with plasma cell dyscrasias and kidney injury have a greater potential to self-associate and to form higher molecular weight aggregates under physiological conditions than clonal FLC from patients without kidney injury. Moreover it has been demonstrated that the injection in mice of clonal FLC derived from patients with renal damage reproduced in the animal the same lesions present in the patient [48–50].

The tropism that some FLC show for the different renal cells seems to be at the basis of the different histopathologic patterns of multiple myeloma and MGRS presentation.

Clonal FLC may present structural and biophysical variations in the variable region (VL) and CDR regions that determine a characteristic toxicity and subsequent damage.

In a series of 11 patients with Fanconi syndrome and histological evidence of light chain proximal tubulopathy, FLC that cause damage were of the κ isotype and presented specific nonpolar or hydrophobic residues in the CDR which determined resistance to proteolysis by cathepsin B [51].

Similarly, FLC inducing cast nephropathy have a particular conformation of the CDR3 region of both κ and λ chains that determines binding to Tamm-Horsfall protein [52].

It has recently been demonstrated that patients with AL amyloidosis present a different amyloidogenic light chain due to genetic rearrangement and somatic hypermutation that determine some biophysical traits correlated with the aggregation propensity and toxicity of light chains, i.e., low fold stability and high protein dynamics [53, 54].

An explanation of the accelerated progression of renal involvement to end-stage renal disease is provided by recent experimental studies.

In vitro studies demonstrated that FLC isolated from the urine of patients affected by multiple myeloma and light chain proteinuria generated hydroxide peroxide and activated the production of monocyte chemoattractant protein 1 (MCP-1), a key chemokine involved in migration and infiltration of monocytes/macrophages [55]. A further insight in the mechanism by which FLC mediate renal injury in MM has recently been given through in vitro and in vivo experiments. Ying W. et al. demonstrated that FLC purified from the urine of patients with MM, light chain proteinuria, and clinical evidence of renal damage induce fibrotic and inflammatory pathways in the kidney; FLC mediate the production of H2O2 through the activation of JAK2/STAT1 signaling and the induction of capsase-1, IL-1β, and TGF-β. Moreover, the authors identified a tryptophan residue within a specific monoclonal FLC that was required for optimal H2O2 production and downstream signaling [56].

On the other hand, the different renal cells could show different responses to the individual clone of FLC. For example, mesangial cells show different intracellular cascade activations in the setting of Al amyloidosis or LCDD; depending on the disease context, mesangial cell can differentiate into macrophage rather than myofibroblast phenotype [57].

Histopathological Lesions in Monoclonal Clone-Related Disorders

The histopathological lesions associated with monoclonal clone-related disorders are wide, involving different structures of the kidney with a specific pattern (Fig. 9.2).

To define the specific renal histological diagnosis, light microscopy and immunofluorescence studies with a full panel of antibodies are required, while electron microscopy is recommended to completely differentiate the histological lesions [58, 59].

Cast nephropathy histologically presents on light microscopy with intratubular casts eosin positive, fractured, and waxy in appearance; the interstitium may present with a lympho-monocyte infiltrate; and cast may be surrounded by multinucleated giant cells. Glomeruli and vessels are not affected directly by the monoclonal disorder until a MGRS pattern is present or there are lesions due to a pre-existing

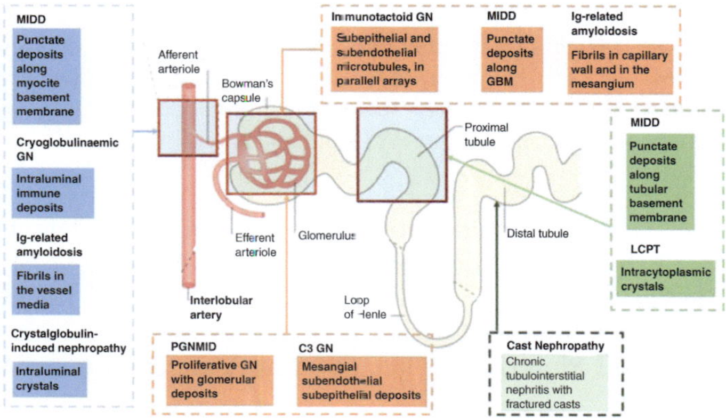

FIGURE 9.2 Schematic representation of localization of the different types of lesions in the kidney

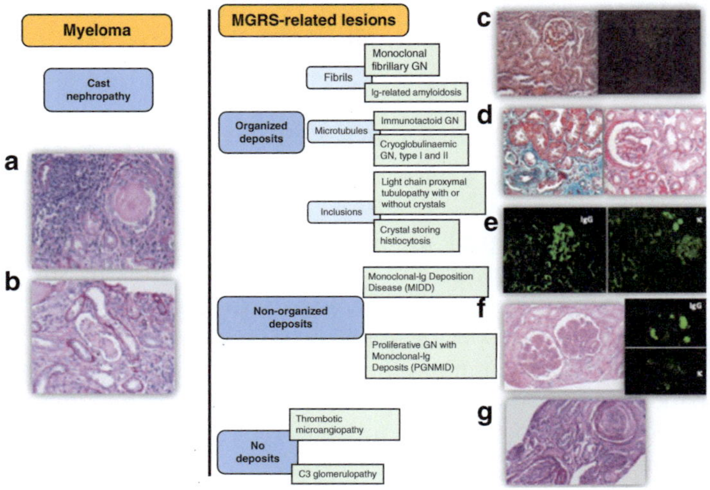

FIGURE 9.3 Categorization of MGRS-associated renal lesions and representative histologic pictures from our histopathologic archive. (**a**, **b**) Cast nephropathy: Periodic acid-Schiff (PAS) staining, magnification 20× (**c**) glomerular amyloidosis. Left: Congo Red staining, magnification 20×. Right: Congo Red staining, magnification 20×, positive for green at polarization, confirming glomerular amyloidosis (**d**) light chain proximal tubulopathy. Left: Masson trichrome staining, magnification 20×. Right: PAS staining, 20×. (**e**) Monoclonal Ig deposition disease (MIDD). Immunofluorescence positive for IgG (left) kappa (right). (**f**) Proliferative GN with monoclonal Ig deposits (PGNMID). Left: hematoxylin eosin staining, magnification 20×, immunofluorescence positive for IgG (top) kappa (bottom). (**g**) Thrombotic microangiopathy. PAS staining, magnification 20×

renal damage. Immunofluorescence staining may demonstrate light chain restriction within the casts (Fig. 9.3).

In 2015, Bridoux et al. described a variety of lesions associated with MGRS, accepted in 2019 by the International Kidney and Monoclonal Gammopathy Research Group [58, 59].

The new classification identifies two main categories of renal lesions, those with organized deposits and the ones with non-organized deposits (Fig. 9.3).

Lesions with Organized Deposits

Deposits of monoclonal immunoglobulin can be organized in fibrils, microtubules, or crystals. Amyloidosis presents with typical non-branching and randomly arranged fibrils, with diameters of 7–12 nm, that involve glomeruli, blood vessels, and the interstitium; fibrils typically stain for Congo red and are composed of light chain, heavy chain, or both. In rare cases the pattern of organized fibrils is that typical of fibrillary glomerulonephritis where fibrils are thicker (10–30 nm) and in the context of a monoclonal gammopathy show a clonal restriction at immunofluorescence. When immunoglobulin deposits arrange in microtubules, i.e., fibrils with hollow centers and large diameters (17–52 nm), the pathological pattern is that of immunotactoid glomerulonephritis and cryoglobulinemic glomerulonephritis, considering only type I and II cryoglobulinemias. The last one presents in the setting of a disease with systemic signs and symptoms, like rashes, peripheral neuropathy, and arthralgias and presents with other typical associated lesions at histology.

Monoclonal light chains can arrange as intracellular inclusions. Usually κ light chain aggregates as crystals inside the cytoplasm and/or the lysosomes of proximal tubular cells, configuring the histopathologic pattern known as light chain proximal tubulopathy (LCPT), and usually presents as complete or partial Fanconi syndrome. LCPT can be the result of deposition of non-crystalline inclusions in proximal tubular cells, mainly distributed inside the lysosomes and constituted by λ monoclonal free light chain; the Fanconi syndrome in this case is less frequent. Rarely light chain crystals can be found both inside tubular cells and in renal histiocytes, configuring the crystal-storing histiocytosis (CSH), whose clinical presentation is widespread systemic, with analogues pattern in different tissues.

Lesions with Non-organized Deposits

Monoclonal immunoglobulin in the form of light chain, heavy chain, or both can deposit inside the basal membrane of glomeruli (GBM) and of tubules configuring the monoclonal immunoglobulin deposition disease (MIDD). When intact immunoglobulin deposit is confined in the different compartments of the glomeruli and is associated with proliferative lesions, the lesion is known as proliferative glomerulonephritis with monoclonal immunoglobulin deposits (PGNMID).

Lesions Without Deposits

In rare cases MGRS can present in the form of C3 glomerulopathy, a rare renal disease with C3 deposition in the glomeruli not/rarely associated with immunoglobulin deposition. In these cases the driving mechanism could be the action of the monoclonal immunoglobulin that acts as a C3 nephritic factor or anti-factor H antibody.

Sometimes MGRS can present as thrombotic microangiopathy (TMA); this endothelial lesion could be the result of the action of the monoclonal immunoglobulin as an autoantibody against a complement regulatory protein. TMA can present associated with polyneuropathy, organomegaly, endocrinopathy, monoclonal gammopathy, and skin changes (POEMS) syndrome.

Therapeutic Insights

Multiple myeloma still has high mortality rate, with a median 5-year survival rate about 50% [60]. The presence of a renal involvement worsens prognosis; in fact, the median survival on dialysis of patients with MM is reported as 18.3 months [5]. Recent advances in MM therapy have improved also renal prognosis. In fact, the reduction of the monoclonal clone with proteasome inhibitors added to the prompt removal of FLC from circulation by apheresis techniques prove some rate of escape from dialysis [10–13]. Moreover, Both proteasome inhibitors and the immunomodulatory drugs lenalidomide and pomalidomide could exert an additional effect on the inflammatory pathways that FLC activate on target organs like the kidney.

The improvement in the understanding of FLC pathogenic structure and its relathionship with some of the clinical and hystological patterns could thoretically lay the foundations for therapy advances.

Kidney Transplant

Renal transplantation is the best renal replacement therapy since the survival benefit it confers to ESRD patients [61]. However, the literature suggest a careful examination of the waiting list patient with a history of multiple myeloma and to consider for transplantation only patients who receive a complete treatment and are on stable complete remission [62, 63]. There is ongoing discussion about the timing of autologous or allogeneic stem cell transplantation (HSCT) in respect to kidney transplantation, with the chance of a living kidney donation from the same HSCT donor [64, 65].

Nevertheless, there are many reports of recurrence of MM or MGRS at different time points after kidney transplant, and, although the median follow-up time is variable, the outcome is not favorable [62, 66–68].

References

1. Tsakiris DJ, Stel VS, Finne P, Fraser E, Heaf J, de Meester J, et al. Incidence and outcome of patients starting renal replacement therapy for end-stage renal disease due to multiple myeloma or light-chain deposit disease: an ERA-EDTA Registry study. Nephrol Dial Transplant [Internet]. 2010 [cited 2019 Nov 10];25(4):1200–6. Available from: http://www.ncbi.nlm.nih.gov/pubmed/20037169.
2. Dimopoulos MA, Kastritis E, Rosinol L, Bladé J, Ludwig H. Pathogenesis and treatment of renal failure in multiple myeloma. Leukemia [Internet]. 2008 [cited 2019 Nov 10];22(8):1485–93. Available from: http://www.nature.com/articles/leu2008131
3. Au EH, Chapman JR, Craig JC, Lim WH, Teixeira-Pinto A, Ullah S, et al. Overall and site-specific cancer mortality in patients on dialysis and after kidney transplant. J Am Soc Nephrol [Internet]. 2019 [cited 2019 Dec 2];30(3). Available from: http://www.ncbi.nlm.nih.gov/pubmed/30765426.
4. Reule S, Sexton DJ, Solid CA, Chen S-C, Foley RN. ESRD due to Multiple Myeloma in the United States, 2001-2010. J Am Soc Nephrol [Internet]. 2016 [cited 2019 Dec 2];27(5):1487–94. Available from: http://www.ncbi.nlm.nih.gov/pubmed/26516209.
5. Decourt A, Gondouin B, Delaroziere JC, Brunet P, Sallée M, Burtey S, et al. Trends in survival and renal recovery in patients with multiple myeloma or light-chain amyloidosis on chronic dialysis. Clin J Am Soc Nephrol [Internet]. 2016 [cited 2019 Dec 2];11(3):431–41. Available from: http://www.ncbi.nlm.nih.gov/pubmed/26728585.
6. Knudsen LM, Hjorth M, Hippe E. Renal failure in multiple myeloma: reversibility and impact on the prognosis. Eur J Haematol [Internet]. 2000 [cited 2019 Nov 10];65(3):175–81. Available from: http://www.ncbi.nlm.nih.gov/pubmed/11007053.
7. Kyle RA, Bergsagel DE. Diagnosis of multiple myeloma. In: Biology and management of multiple myeloma [Internet]. Totowa, NJ: Humana Press; 2004 [cited 2019 Nov 10]. p. 1–11. Available from: http://link.springer.com/10.1007/978-1-59259-817-5_1
8. Heher EC, Goes NB, Spitzer TR, Raje NS, Humphreys BD, Anderson KC, et al. Kidney disease associated with plasma cell dyscrasias. Blood [Internet]. 2010 [cited 2019 Nov 10];116(9):1397–404. Available from: http://www.ncbi.nlm.nih.gov/pubmed/20462963.

9. Bladé J, Fernández-Llama P, Bosch F, Montolíu J, Lens XM, Montoto S, et al. Renal failure in multiple myeloma. Arch Intern Med [Internet]. 1998 [cited 2019 Nov 10];158(17):1889. Available from: http://archinte.jamanetwork.com/article.aspx?doi=10.1001/archinte.158.17.1889
10. Dimopoulos MA, Sonneveld P, Leung N, Merlini G, Ludwig H, Kastritis E, et al. International myeloma working group recommendations for the diagnosis and management of myeloma-related renal impairment. J Clin Oncol [Internet]. 2016 [cited 2019 Nov 10];34(13):1544–57. Available from: http://ascopubs.org/doi/10.1200/JCO.2015.65.0044
11. Hutchison CA, Cockwell P, Stringer S, Bradwell A, Cook M, Gertz MA, et al. Early reduction of serum-free light chains associates with renal recovery in myeloma kidney. J Am Soc Nephrol [Internet]. 2011 [cited 2019 Nov 10];22(6):1129–36. Available from: http://www.jasn.org/lookup/doi/10.1681/ASN.2010080857
12. Donati G, Zappulo F, Croci Chiocchini AL, Comai G, Zamagni E, La Manna G. Early use of PEPA dialyzer for light chains removal and for the recovery from myeloma cast nephropathy: A case report. Hemodial Int [Internet]. 2019 [cited 2019 Dec 7];23(3):E97–9. Available from: http://doi.wiley.com/10.1111/hdi.12733
13. Hogan JJ, Weiss BM. Bridging the divide: an onco-nephrologic approach to the monoclonal gammopathies of renal significance. Clin J Am Soc Nephrol [Internet]. 2016 [cited 2019 Nov 11];11(9):1681–91. Available from: http://cjasn.asnjournals.org/lookup/doi/10.2215/CJN.03160316
14. Paueksakon P, Revelo MP, Horn RG, Shappell S, Fogo AB. Monoclonal gammopathy: significance sand possible causality in renal disease. Am J Kidney Dis [Internet]. 2003 [cited 2019 Nov 11];42(1):87–95. Available from: http://www.ncbi.nlm.nih.gov/pubmed/12830460.
15. Leung N, Bridoux F, Hutchison CA, Nasr SH, Cockwell P, Fermand J-P, et al. Monoclonal gammopathy of renal significance: when MGUS is no longer undetermined or insignificant. Blood [Internet]. 2012 [cited 2019 Nov 11];120(22):4292–5. Available from: http://www.ncbi.nlm.nih.gov/pubmed/23047823.
16. Vignon M, Javaugue V, Alexander MP, El-Karoui K, Karras A, Roos-Weil D, et al. Current anti-myeloma therapies in renal manifestations of monoclonal light chain-associated Fanconi syndrome: a retrospective series of 49 patients. Leukemia [Internet]. 2017 [cited 2019 Nov 11];31(1):123–9. Available from: http://www.nature.com/articles/leu2016195

17. Sayed RH, Wechalekar AD, Gilbertson JA, Bass P, Mahmood S, Sachchithanantham S, et al. Natural history and outcome of light chain deposition disease. Blood [Internet]. 2015 [cited 2019 Nov 11];126(26):2805–10. Available from: https://ashpublications.org/blood/article/126/26/2805/34774/Natural-history-and-outcome-of-light-chain
18. Hassoun H, Flombaum C, D'Agati VD, Rafferty BT, Cohen A, Klimek VM, et al. High-dose melphalan and auto-SCT in patients with monoclonal Ig deposition disease. Bone Marrow Transplant [Internet]. 2008 [cited 2019 Nov 11];42(6):405–12. Available from: http://www.nature.com/articles/bmt2008179
19. Cohen C, Royer B, Javaugue V, Szalat R, El Karoui K, Caulier A, et al. Bortezomib produces high hematological response rates with prolonged renal survival in monoclonal immunoglobulin deposition disease. Kidney Int [Internet]. 2015 [cited 2019 Nov 11];88(5):1135–43. Available from: https://linkinghub.elsevier.com/retrieve/pii/S0085253815609930
20. Chauvet S, Frémeaux-Bacchi V, Petitprez F, Karras A, Daniel L, Burtey S, et al. Treatment of B-cell disorder improves renal outcome of patients with monoclonal gammopathy-associated C3 glomerulopathy. Blood [Internet]. 2017 [cited 2019 Nov 11];129(11):1437–47. Available from: https://ashpublications.org/blood/article/129/11/1437/35927/Treatment-of-Bcell-disorder-improves-renal-outcome
21. Nasr SH, Satoskar A, Markowitz GS, Valeri AM, Appel GB, Stokes MB, et al. Proliferative glomerulonephritis with monoclonal IgG deposits. J Am Soc Nephrol [Internet]. 2009 [cited 2019 Nov 11];20(9):2055–64. Available from: http://www.jasn.org/lookup/doi/10.1681/ASN.2009010110
22. Bridoux F, Hugue V, Coldefy O, Goujon J-M, Bauwens M, Sechet A, et al. Fibrillary glomerulonephritis and immunotactoid (microtubular) glomerulopathy are associated with distinct immunologic features. Kidney Int [Internet]. 2002 [cited 2019 Nov 11];62(5):1764–75. Available from: https://linkinghub.elsevier.com/retrieve/pii/S0085253815487344
23. Gertz MA, Leung N, Lacy MQ, Dispenzieri A, Zeldenrust SR, Hayman SR, et al. Clinical outcome of immunoglobulin light chain amyloidosis affecting the kidney. Nephrol Dial Transplant [Internet]. 2009 [cited 2019 Nov 11];24(10):3132–7. Available from: https://academic.oup.com/ndt/article-lookup/doi/10.1093/ndt/gfp201
24. National Comprehensive Cancer Network. National Comprehensive Cancer Network. NCCN Clinical Practice

Guidelines in Oncology, Multiple Myeloma. Version 3 2019 [Internet]. Available from: http://www.nccn.org/professionals/physician_gls/pdf/myeloma.pdf.
25. Nasr SH, Valeri AM, Sethi S, Fidler ME, Cornell LD, Gertz MA, et al. Clinicopathologic correlations in multiple myeloma: a case series of 190 patients with kidney biopsies. Am J Kidney Dis [Internet]. 2012 [cited 2019 Dec 4];59(6):786–94. Available from: https //linkinghub.elsevier.com/retrieve/pii/S0272638612001357
26. Sethi S, Rajkumar SV, D'Agati VD. The complexity and heterogeneity of monoclonal immunoglobulin-associated renal diseases. J Am Soc Nephrol [Internet]. 2018 [cited 2019 Dec 2];29(7):1810–23. Available from: http://www.ncbi.nlm.nih.gov/pubmed/29703839.
27. Akilesh S, Christianson GJ, Roopenian DC, Shaw AS. Neonatal FcR expression in bone marrow-derived cells functions to protect serum IgG from catabolism. J Immunol [Internet]. 2007 [cited 2019 Nov 9];179(7):4580–8. Available from: http://www.jimmunol.org/lookup/doi/10.4049/jimmunol.179.7.4580
28. Kim J, Hayton WL, Robinson JM, Anderson CL. Kinetics of FcRn-mediated recycling of IgG and albumin in human: pathophysiology and therapeutic implications using a simplified mechanism-based model. Clin Immunol [Internet]. 2007 [cited 2019 Nov 9];122(2):146–55. Available from: https://linkinghub.elsevier.com/retrieve/pii/S1521661606008722
29. Waldmann TA, Strober W. Metabolism of immunoglobulins. In: Progress in allergy [Internet]. 1969 [cited 2019 Nov 9]. p. 1–110. Available from: http://www.ncbi.nlm.nih.gov/pubmed/4186070.
30. Hogan JJ, Alexander MP, Leung N. Dysproteinemia and the kidney: core curriculum 2019. Am J Kidney Dis [Internet]. 2019 [cited 2019 Sep 28]; Available from: https://linkinghub.elsevier.com/retrieve/pii/S027263861930798X
31. The Binding Site Group Ltd. The biology of immunoglobulins | Wikilite [Internet]. [cited 2019 Nov 9]. Available from: http://www.wikilite.com/the-biology-of-immunoglobulins
32. Waldmann TA, Strober W, Mogielnicki RP. The renal handling of low molecular weight proteins. J Clin Invest [Internet]. 1972 [cited 2019 Nov 9];51(8):2162–74. Available from: http://www.ncbi.nlm.nih.gov/pubmed/5054468.
33. Hutchison CA, Cockwell P, Reid S, Chandler K, Mead GP, Harrison J, et al. Efficient removal of immunoglobulin free light chains by hemodialysis for multiple myeloma: *In Vitro* and *In Vivo* studies. J Am Soc Nephrol [Internet]. 2007 [cited 2019 Nov

9];18(3):886–95. Available from: http://www.ncbi.nlm.nih.gov/pubmed/17229909.
34. Katzmann JA, Clark RJ, Abraham RS, Bryant S, Lymp JF, Bradwell AR, et al. Serum reference intervals and diagnostic ranges for free kappa and free lambda immunoglobulin light chains: relative sensitivity for detection of monoclonal light chains. Clin Chem [Internet]. 2002 [cited 2019 Nov 9];48(9):1437–44. Available from: http://www.ncbi.nlm.nih.gov/pubmed/12194920.
35. Wochner RD, Strober W, Waldmann TA. The role of the kidney in the catabolism of Bence Jones proteins and immunoglobulin fragments. J Exp Med [Internet]. 1967 [cited 2019 Nov 9];126(2):207–21. Available from: http://www.jem.org/cgi/doi/10.1084/jem.126.2.207
36. Hutchison CA, Harding S, Hewins P, Mead GP, Townsend J, Bradwell AR, et al. Quantitative assessment of serum and urinary polyclonal free light chains in patients with chronic kidney disease. Clin J Am Soc Nephrol [Internet]. 2008 [cited 2019 Nov 9];3(6):1684–90. Available from: http://www.ncbi.nlm.nih.gov/pubmed/18945993.
37. Solomon A, Waldmann TA, Fahey JL, McFarlane AS. Metabolism of Bence Jones Proteins*. J Clin Invest [Internet]. 1964 [cited 2019 Nov 9];43(1):103–17. Available from: http://www.ncbi.nlm.nih.gov/pubmed/14105221.
38. Miettinen TA, Kekki M. Effect of impaired hepatic and renal function on [131]bence jones protein catabolism in human subjects. Clin Chim Acta [Internet]. 1967 [cited 2019 Nov 9];18(3):395–407. Available from: https://www.sciencedirect.com/science/article/abs/pii/0009898167900368
39. Hutchison CA, Basnayake K, Cockwell P. Serum free light chain assessment in monoclonal gammopathy and kidney disease. Nat Rev Nephrol [Internet]. 2009 [cited 2019 Nov 9];5(11):621–8. Available from: http://www.ncbi.nlm.nih.gov/pubmed/19786994.
40. Christensen EI, Birn H, Storm T, Weyer K, Nielsen R. Endocytic receptors in the renal proximal tubule. Physiology [Internet]. 2012 [cited 2019 Nov 9];27(4):223–36. Available from: http://www.ncbi.nlm.nih.gov/pubmed/22875453.
41. Maack T, Johnson V, Kau ST, Figueiredo J, Sigulem D. Renal filtration, transport, and metabolism of low-molecular-weight proteins: a review. Kidney Int [Internet]. 1979 [cited 2019 Nov 9];16(3):251–70. Available from: http://www.ncbi.nlm.nih.gov/pubmed/393891.
42. Brenner BM, Taal MW, Chertow GM, Marsden PA, Skorecki K. The kidney. Vol. 1.

43. American Society of Biological Chemists, Rockefeller Institute for Medical Research, American Society for Biochemistry and Molecular Biology. The Journal of biological chemistry. [Internet]. American Society for Biochemistry and Molecular Biology; [cited 2019 Nov 9]. Available from: http://www.jbc.org/content/244/16/4299?ijkey=4ed6fe426380c05c283833e4a77925a635a16301&keytype2=tf_ipsecsha
44. Clyne DH, Pollak VE. Renal Handling and Pathophysiology of Bence Jones Proteins1. In Karger Publishers; 1981 [cited 2019 Nov 9]. p. 78–87. Available from: https://www.karger.com/Article/FullText/395232
45. Christensen EI, Birn H. Megalin and cubilin: synergistic endocytic receptors in renal proximal tubule. Am J Physiol Physiol [Internet]. 2001 cited 2019 Nov 9];280(4):F562–73. Available from: http://www.ncbi.nlm.nih.gov/pubmed/11249847.
46. Mead GP, Carr-Smith HD, Drayson MT, Morgan GJ, Child JA, Bradwell AR. Serum free light chains for monitoring multiple myeloma. Br J Haematol [Internet]. 2004 [cited 2019 Nov 9];126(3):348–54. Available from: http://doi.wiley.com/10.1111/j.1365-2141 2004.05045.x
47. Sanders PW. SCIENCE IN RENAL MEDICINE Mechanisms of Light Chain Injury along the Tubular Nephron. J Am Soc Nephrol [Internet]. 2012 [cited 2019 Nov 9];23:1777–81. Available from: www.jasn.org
48. Solomon A, Weiss DT, Kattine AA. Nephrotoxic potential of Bence Jones proteins. N Engl J Med [Internet]. 1991 [cited 2019 Nov 11];324(26):1845–51. Available from: http://www.nejm.org/doi/abs/10.1056/NEJM199106273242603
49. Myatt EA, Westholm FA, Weiss DT, Solomon A, Schiffer M, Stevens FJ. Pathogenic potential of human monoclonal immunoglobulin light chains: relationship of in vitro aggregation to in vivo organ deposition. Proc Natl Acad Sci [Internet]. 1994 [cited 2019 Nov 11];91(8):3034–8. Available from: http://www.ncbi.nlm.nih.gov/pubmed/8159701.
50. Sirac C, Herrera GA, Sanders PW, Batuman V, Bender S, Ayala M V, et al. Animal models of monoclonal immunoglobulin-related renal diseases. Nat Rev Nephrol [Internet]. 2018 [cited 2019 Nov 11];14(4):246–64. Available from: http://www.nature.com/articles/nrneph.2018.8
51. Messiaen T, Deret S, Mougenot B, Bridoux F, Dequiedt P, Dion JJ, et al. Adult Fanconi syndrome secondary to light chain gammopathy. Clinicopathologic heterogeneity and unusual features in 11 patients. Medicine (Baltimore) [Internet]. 2000 [cited 2019

Dec 7];79(3):135–54. Available from: http://www.ncbi.nlm.nih.gov/pubmed/10844934.

52. Ying WZ, Sanders PW. Mapping the binding domain of immunoglobulin light chains for Tamm-Horsfall protein. Am J Pathol [Internet]. 2001 [cited 2019 Dec 7];158(5):1859–66. Available from: https://linkinghub.elsevier.com/retrieve/pii/S0002944010641429
53. Oberti L, Maritan M, Rognoni P, Barbiroli A, Lavatelli F, Russo R, et al. The concurrency of several biophysical traits links immunoglobulin light chains with toxicity in AL amyloidosis. Amyloid [Internet]. 2019 [cited 2019 Dec 7];26(sup1):107–8. Available from: http://www.ncbi.nlm.nih.gov/pubmed/31343357.
54. Oberti L, Rognoni P, Barbiroli A, Lavatelli F, Russo R, Maritan M, et al. Concurrent structural and biophysical traits link with immunoglobulin light chains amyloid propensity. Sci Rep [Internet]. 2017 [cited 2019 Dec 7];7(1):16809. Available from: http://www.ncbi.nlm.nih.gov/pubmed/29196671.
55. Wang P-X, Sanders PW. Immunoglobulin light chains generate hydrogen peroxide. J Am Soc Nephrol [Internet]. 2007 [cited 2019 Dec 7];18(4):1239–45. Available from: http://www.jasn.org/lookup/doi/10.1681/ASN.2006111299
56. Ying W-Z, Li X, Rangarajan S, Feng W, Curtis LM, Sanders PW. Immunoglobulin light chains generate proinflammatory and profibrotic kidney injury. J Clin Invest [Internet]. 2019 [cited 2019 Nov 9];129(7):2792–806. Available from: http://www.ncbi.nlm.nih.gov/pubmed/31205024.
57. Basnayake K, Stringer SJ, Hutchison CA, Cockwell P. The biology of immunoglobulin free light chains and kidney injury. Kidney Int [Internet]. 2011 [cited 2019 Nov 9];79(12):1289–301. Available from: http://www.ncbi.nlm.nih.gov/pubmed/21490587.
58. Leung N, Bridoux F, Batuman V, Chaidos A, Cockwell P, D'Agati VD, et al. The evaluation of monoclonal gammopathy of renal significance: a consensus report of the International Kidney and Monoclonal Gammopathy Research Group. Nat Rev Nephrol [Internet]. 2019 [cited 2019 Nov 11];15(1):45–59. Available from: http://www.ncbi.nlm.nih.gov/pubmed/30510265.
59. Bridoux F, Leung N, Hutchison CA, Touchard G, Sethi S, Fermand J-P, et al. Diagnosis of monoclonal gammopathy of renal significance. Kidney Int [Internet]. 2015 [cited 2019 Nov 11];87(4):698–711. Available from: http://www.ncbi.nlm.nih.gov/pubmed/25607108.

60. American Cancer Society. Cancer Facts & Figures 2018. Available from: https://www.cancer.org/content/dam/cancer-org/research/cancer-facts-and-statistics/annual-cancer-facts-and-figures/2018/cancer-facts-and-figures-2018.pdf
61. United States Renal Data System (USRDS). v2 CH6 Transplantation [Internet]. [cited 2019 Dec 7]. Available from: https://www.usrds.org/2018/view/v2_06.aspx
62. Cowan AJ, Johnson CK, Libby EN. Plasma cell diseases and organ transplant: A comprehensive review. Am J Transplant [Internet]. 2018 [cited 2019 Dec 7];18(5):1046–58. Available from: http://doi.wiley.com/10.1111/ajt.14731
63. Kdigo clinical practice guideline on the evaluation and management of candidates for kidney transplantation public review draft [Internet]. 2018 [cited 2019 Dec 7]. Available from: https://kdigo.org/wp-content/uploads/2018/08/KDIGO-Txp-Candidate-GL-Public-Review-Draft-Oct-22.pdf
64. Baraldi O, Grandinetti V, Donati G, Comai G, Battaglino G, Cuna V, et al. Hematopoietic cell and renal transplantation in plasma cell dyscrasia patients. Cell Transplant [Internet]. 2016 [cited 2019 Dec 7];25(6):995–1005. Available from: http://journals.sagepub.com/doi/full/10.3727/096368915X688560
65. Chen Y-B, Elias N, Heher E, McCune JS, Collier K, Li S, et al. Haploidentical hematopoietic cell and kidney transplantation for hematological malignancies and end-stage renal failure. Blood [Internet]. 2019 [cited 2019 Dec 7];134(2):211–5. Available from: http://www.ncbi.nlm.nih.gov/pubmed/31151984.
66. Lum EL, Bunnapradist S. Current opinions in nephrology and hypertension. Curr Opin Nephrol Hypertens [Internet]. 2019 [cited 2019 Dec 7];28(6):573–80. Available from: http://www.ncbi.nlm.nih.gov/pubmed/31403474.
67. Moog P, Jost PJ, Büttner-Herold M. Eculizumab as salvage therapy for recurrent monoclonal gammopathy-induced C3 glomerulopathy in a kidney allograft. BMC Nephrol [Internet]. 2018 [cited 2019 Dec 7];19(1):106. Available from: https://bmcnephrol.biomedcentral.com/articles/10.1186/s12882-018-0904-7
68. Angel-Korman A, Stern L, Sarosiek S, Sloan JM, Doros G, Sanchorawala V, et al. Long-term outcome of kidney transplantation in AL amyloidosis. Kidney Int [Internet]. 2019 [cited 2019 Dec 7];95(2):405–11. Available from: https://linkinghub.elsevier.com/retrieve/pii/S0085253818307749

Chapter 10
Treatment of Multiple Myeloma with Kidney Involvement

Mark A. Cook

Evidence Base

It is a regrettable fact that despite the fact that just under 4% of patients with newly diagnosed myeloma present with acute kidney injury (AKI) severe enough to require dialysis and up to 40% have some degree of renal impairment (RI), they are frequently excluded from clinical trials, where entry criteria usually require an estimated glomerular filtration rate (eGFR) of 30, 40 or 50 ml/min. Indeed, a search of the clinicaltrials.gov database using the terms 'myeloma' and 'renal impairment' (accessed 25 September 2019, spanning the dates 2003 to date of accession) identifies 30 interventional trials targeting patients with myeloma and RI – if all fully

M. A. Cook (✉)
Centre for Clinical Haematology, Queen Elizabeth Hospital Birmingham and Institute of Cancer and Genomic Sciences, University of Birmingham, Birmingham, UK
e-mail: mark.cook@uhb.nhs.uk

E. Zamagni (ed.), *Management of Bone Disease and Kidney Failure in Multiple Myeloma*,
https://doi.org/10.1007/978-3-030-63662-3_10

recruit, then the total number of patients will only be 2205. The search term 'myeloma' returns 2550 studies.

We are therefore left with an evidence base that is very limited, primarily about therapeutic interventions and very rarely about the supportive care required in this patient group. Thus, advice on how to manage these patients requires expert opinion based as much on experience as on the evidence available.

General Principles

Patients with acute kidney injury (AKI) due to undiagnosed myeloma do not necessarily present to the haematologist first. Patients will often present to general physicians or to nephrologists directly – and it is the subsequent path of diagnostics that ultimately brings the patient to the care of the haematologist. It is thus crucial that the clinicians most likely to be involved in this pathway understand the importance of their role in the successful outcome for such patients, expediting the appropriate investigations such as measurement of serum free light chains (FLCs) to secure an early diagnosis. For those patients presenting with AKI requiring dialysis support, there is a window of approximately 6 weeks in which the renal lesion may be reversed and the patient may become free from dialysis [1]. Indeed, freedom from dialysis is highly dependent on the speedy institution of treatment and a response within 21 days [2]. It is imperative that such patients are managed within a multidisciplinary environment with engaged nephrologists, haematologists and pathologists working together efficiently to make a diagnosis and institute a management plan.

There is ample evidence that renal recovery (particularly becoming free from dialysis) is associated with improved survival [3], and there is a clear quality of life benefit to not being on dialysis. Any patient presenting with AKI secondary to myeloma should be regarded as a medical emergency. Successful outcome depends on a three-pronged approach –

prompt assessment and removal of precipitating factors, high-quality supportive care and rapid reduction in serum FLC levels by the use of highly effective anti-myeloma therapy.

Prompt Assessment

Firstly, a thorough clinical evaluation and removal of precipitating factors are mandated. A complete drug history should be taken, looking for medications that can be associated with worsening of renal function such as non-steroidal anti-inflammatory drugs (NSAIDs). It is important therefore that the patient is asked about over-the-counter medication and herbal/complementary medication, as well as a review of their prescribed medication. Implicated medications should be stopped, including loop diuretics which can worsen cast nephropathy [4] and NSAIDs.

High-Quality Supportive Care

Secondly, the patient should be evaluated for any evidence of infection/sepsis and managed accordingly with antibiotics if detected. Hypercalcaemia and secondary dehydration should be looked for as potentially reversible causes of RI, with accurate evaluation of fluid balance and institution of intravenous fluids in those considered volume-depleted. The dogma of ensuring adequate fluid intake (of 3 L/day) originates in the UK MRC Myeloma IV study in which patients presenting with RI were randomised to advice on fluid intake of 3 L/day or not. There was a higher rate of renal recovery and overall survival was significantly higher in the 3 L/day arm [5].

Rapid Reduction in Circulating Serum FLC Levels

The prime aim of treatment is to reduce the circulating level of serum FLCs, as this will reduce the ongoing formation of intraluminal waxy casts, thus raising the prospect of reversal of RI. There is some evidence that in severe cast nephropathy where renal replacement therapy is required, the 'window of opportunity' to reverse the RI is in the region of 6 weeks. Another principle established in modelling and early-phase clinical studies is that the likelihood of renal recovery is dependent on the reduction in serum FLC level by as early as day 21. It is thus imperative, once the diagnosis of renal failure secondary to myeloma is confirmed, to commence anti-myeloma therapy.

Mechanical Removal of Circulating Free Light Chains

What of mechanical removal of circulating FLCs? Intuitively, if the level of circulating FLCs can be kept below the level of 500 mg/L (at which point the proximal tubular mechanism is saturated and free light chains enter the renal collecting system), then this raises the prospect of permitting earlier renal recovery, whilst waiting for the anti-myeloma therapy to cause enough tumour kill to significantly reduce light chain production. The two main methods of mechanical removal are plasma exchange and high cut-off (HCO) dialysis.

Plasma Exchange

Plasma exchange has been a mainstay of the management of hyperviscosity related to plasma cell disorders for over half a century. Johnson and colleagues published the outcomes of a small-scale study in patients with myeloma and progressive renal failure [6]. Patients were randomised to forced diuresis and chemotherapy or forced diuresis, chemotherapy and plasmapheresis. Whilst chemotherapy, plasmapheresis and forced diuresis together more effectively lowered the serum myeloma protein value, the only determinant of outcome was the severity of myeloma cast formation on renal biopsy. Subsequent small studies (Zucchelli et al. [7], Moist et al. [8])

suggested that plasma exchange may offer a benefit in combination with treating the underlying myeloma – that benefit being either avoidance of dialysis or, if dialysis-dependent, subsequent freedom from dialysis. These were small studies – one a retrospective chart review [8]. Nevertheless, there was a small but growing body of opinion that there may well be a benefit in terms of outcome if plasma exchange were to be added to the initial regimen of treatment for these patients. A larger study by Clark et al. randomised patients between conventional therapy plus 5–7 plasma exchanges for 10 days or conventional therapy alone [9]. The primary outcome was a composite measure of death, dialysis dependence or a GFR of <30 mL/min per 1.73m^2. Ninety-six patients were evaluable. The primary composite end point occurred in 33 out of 57 patients in the plasma exchange group (57.9%) and 27 out of 39 (69.2%) in the control group – the conclusion being that 5–7 plasma exchanges did not substantially reduce the composite outcome. This study was limited by the lack of ability to measure FLCs and the absence of renal biopsy on study entry – thus neither the nature of the renal lesion nor the degree of response could be accurately determined.

Drayson and colleagues have reported – in abstract form only – the findings of the UK NCRI MyEloma RI Trial (MERIT) in which patients with newly diagnosed myeloma and acute renal failure were randomised to chemotherapy alone or chemotherapy and plasma exchange (7 treatments in total over 14 days, with 4 of those in the first 7 days) [10]. Treatment of myeloma was initiated with pulsed dexamethasone (40 mg daily on days 1–4 and 9–12). Treatment was then continued with VAD (vincristine, Adriamycin and dexamethasone) for 4 cycles (amended to physician's choice in 2006). A total of 78 patients were randomised at the time of presentation in 2012. There was no statistical difference between the two groups in terms of alive and dialysis-independent at day 100 (28.9% in the plasma exchange group vs 25% in the control group). There was no difference in overall survival between the two arms. However, what this study demonstrated was that, independent of treatment, the patients who were alive and dialysis-independent at day 100 had significantly lower FLC levels than those patients who remained dialysis-dependent or had died. So whilst plasma exchange cannot be recommended as a standard of care in this patient group, the concept that reduction in FLC level is the key to renal recovery remains the mainstay of the present approach to this patient group.

High Cut-Off (HCO) Dialysis

As evidenced above, plasma exchange had been regarded as the likeliest way to mechanically reduce the level of circulating FLC, primarily because the pore size in conventional dialysis filters did not permit the removal of significant amounts of FLC during haemodialysis (HD). This changed with the development of the high cut-off dialyser (HCO-1100 Gambro). FLCs exist as either a monomer kappa (κ) 25 kDa in size or as a dimer lambda (λ) 50 kDa in size. HCO dialysers are highly permeable to low molecular weight proteins of up to 50 kDa, raising the possibility of efficient removal of circulating FLCs by this method. Mathematical modelling based on *in vitro* experiments using model systems demonstrated that FLC clearance of >50% can be achieved with HCO dialysis filters [11]. The model also showed that effective anti-myeloma therapy combined with HCO dialysis could, in theory, lead to a rapid normalisation of circulating FLCs and increase the potential for renal recovery. Early clinical cases appeared to corroborate this, with over 50% of patients becoming independent of dialysis compared to a historical rate of less than 20%. Subsequently, two randomised phase 2 trials have tested the utility of the addition of HCO dialysis techniques to effective chemotherapy.

In the MYRE study, Bridoux and colleagues recruited patients with biopsy-proven cast nephropathy [12]. Those requiring HD were entered into a randomised part of the MYRE study evaluating HCO dialysis (50 patients) compared with conventional HD (48 patients). All patients received a combination of bortezomib (1.3 mg/m^2 days 1, 4, 8 and 11 of a 21 day cycle) and dexamethasone (20 mg on days 1–2, 4–5, 8–9 and 11–12). Patients aged over 70 had the frequency of bortezomib dropped to once weekly for a 28 day cycle after cycle 1. After the third cycle, cyclophosphamide (750 mg/m^2 on day 1) was added in to non-responding patients to try and improve the likelihood of response. Both groups had eight HD sessions planned in the first 10 days. They could receive three additional weekly HD sessions if required using the same dialyser until the completion of cycle 3. The primary end point was independence of HD at 3 months after randomisation. Withdrawal of HD was physician determined as per local practice. Secondary end points included myeloma response, EFS, RFS and OS. The independence from dialysis rate at 3 months was 41.3% in the HCO group and 33.3% in the conventional HD group ($p = 0.42$). Within the secondary end points, there were some interesting findings. Cumulative independence of HD at 6 months was significantly different (56.5% for HCO versus 35.4% for conventional HD, $p = 0.04$), improving further by 12 months (60.9% and 37.5% respectively, $p = 0.02$). Better haematologic responses were seen in the HCO group at 3 months, but this did not translate into an improved rate of VGPR or better. Twenty-eight per cent of patients in the HCO group and 23% of patients in the conventional HD group had cyclophosphamide added in at a median of 4.4 months and 4.1 months, respectively. By 6 months, the VGPR or better rate in the HCO group was 69.6% versus 47.9% ($p = 0.03$), although it should be borne in mind that the conventional HD group had a higher percentage of high-risk patients (by FISH, 26% for conventional HD vs 15% for HCO). Achieving a serum FLC level of less than 500 mg/L was shown to be an independent predictive factor of HD independence at 12 months, as was the use of the HCO filter.

In the EuLITE study, Hutchison and colleagues randomised 90 patients with biopsy-proven cast nephropathy requiring HD to HCO dialysis or conventional HD [13]. HCO dialysis was performed using two HCO-1100 dialysers in series (giving a surface area of 2.2 m², compared to a single 2.1 m² dialyser used in the MYRE study). All patients received the same chemotherapy, a modified PAD regimen (bortezomib 1 mg/m² on days 1, 4, 8 and 11 of a 21 day cycle), doxorubicin (9 mg/m² on days 1 and 4 of the 21 day cycle) and dexamethasone (40 mg daily days 1–4, 8–11 and 15–18 for the first 21 day cycle and days 1–4 only on subsequent cycles). The primary end point was independence of dialysis at 3 months. The rate at 3 months was 55.8% in the HCO group and 51.1% in the conventional HD group ($p = 0.811$). In total, 58.1% in the HCO group and 66% in the conventional HD group became independent of HD. There was no significant difference in the time to independence of HD. When adjusted by age category at randomisation, the hazard ratio for death was 2.63 (CI, 1.13–6.16; $p = 0.026$) in the HCO arm compared to the control arm, although there was no statistically significant single reason for the increased mortality seen. Interestingly, there was an increased incidence of respiratory infections seen in the HCO arm (12 vs 2, $p = 0.0082$). Response rates at 6 months were not statistically different but at 12 months were significantly better in the control arm (RR 0.62; CI, 0.41–0.92; $p = 0.022$).

So what can we conclude from the MYRE and EuLITE studies? There are clearly design differences. The EuLITE authors calculate that HCO patients in EuLITE had 40% greater treatment length with HCO-HD than their equivalent in MYRE in the first 10 days – yet showed no benefit from this intervention. There is a distinct difference between the chemotherapy regimens used – in EuLITE a triplet with intense steroid dosing in cycle 1 (PAD) and in MYRE a doublet (bortezomib/dexamethasone). Within 4–6 days, median levels of FLCs were around 50% of pretreatment levels in both arms of EuLITE, indicating a highly effective chemotherapeutic impact. FLC levels fell further – to 20% of pretreatment levels by days 10–12 and 10% by days 20–22. This is the likeliest explanation for renal recovery of such high rates in both arms of the study – and the rates seen are higher than those seen in MYRE at 3 months. It is less easy to explain the higher mortality in the HCO arm in EuLITE – although the extended dialysis required significant albumin replacement, a marker of overall protein loss which could also include cytokines, growth factors and other immune regulators. In conclusion, the argument for mechanical removal of excess light chains cannot be supported by the data to date, and as chemotherapy becomes more effective with higher response rates and speed of response, the likelihood of mechanical removal having a role is increasingly unlikely.

Chemotherapeutic Approach

The aim of chemotherapy is simple in the situation of renal failure due to myeloma – reduce the myeloma burden as quickly as possible, thereby reducing the light chain burden below 500 mg/L – thought to be the critical level at which cast formation begins within the tubular lumen. A summary of drugs currently available is in Table 10.1, along with dose adjustments where information is available. The backbone to all modern therapeutic regimens is dexamethasone, a potent corticosteroid. Its effectiveness was first described in combination by Barlogie et al. [14], with a subsequent paper showing that the majority of benefit from the VAD (vincristine, Adriamycin, dexamethasone) regimen was from the dexamethasone [15]. The era of the novel agents began with the introduction of thalidomide, soon followed by bortezomib and lenalidomide. All of these were shown to be highly effective in combination with dexamethasone. There has subsequently been a rapid increase in the number of new agents achieving marketing authorisation in the treatment of myeloma. With variations between drugs (even in the same class) as to how well they are tolerated in RI, it is important to understand the pharmacokinetics of the drugs to be used in any given patient, with appropriate dose adjustments made. As indicated at the beginning of the chapter, patients with severe RI are nearly always excluded from clinical trials – certainly those performed to achieve marketing authori-

TABLE 10.1 Renal impairment and drugs used in the treatment of myeloma

Drug class	Agent	Dose adjustment in renal impairment	Additional comments	Key references
Steroid	Dexamethasone	None		[10]
	Prednisolone	None		
Alkylator	Cyclophosphamide	CrCl <10 mL/min – 50% reduction		[61]
	High-dose melphalan	30% reduction in autologous stem cell transplantation if CrCl <50 mL/min		[54]
	Oral melphalan	CrCl 45–60 mL/min – 85% of full dose CrCl 30–45 mL/min – 75% of full dose CrCl 10–30 mL/min – 70% of full dose CrCl <10 mL/min – 50% of full dose		[61]
	Bendamustine	Unclear – case reports of effective use		[31, 32]
Proteasome inhibitor	Bortezomib	None		[18, 19, 21]
	Carfilzomib			[23]

	Ixazomib	Reduce to 3 mg once weekly if eGFR <30 mL/min		[26]
Immunomodulatory	Thalidomide	None	Reports of hyperkalaemia	[27]
	Lenalidomide	CrCl 30–49 mL/min – 10 mg od CrCL<30 mL/min not on dialysis – 7.5 mg od or 15 mg eod ESRD requiring dialysis – 5 mg od	Administer dose after dialysis	[34, 62]
	Pomalidomide	None		[37]
Monoclonal antibody	Daratumumab	None	Infusional volume needs to be carefully managed in patients on haemodialysis	[47]
	Elotuzumab	None		[50]
HDAC inhibitor	Panobinostat	None	Used in combination with bortezomib and dexamethasone – reduction of bortezomib to once weekly reduces AEs	[41]

CrCl creatinine clearance, *eGFR* estimated GFR, *ESRD* end stage renal disease, *od* once daily, *eod* every other day sation. Unfortunately, this means that the clinician is often dependent on subgroup analyses of such studies or small-scale pharmacokinetic (PK)/pharmacodynamic studies to try and choose a combination that is highly effective but at the same time has minimal toxicity.

Single Agent Dexamethasone

Dexamethasone by itself has utility in the emergency situation, as it is accessible 24 hours a day in most hospital environments. Thus a patient presenting with severe AKI in the context of myeloma can be commenced on dexamethasone straight away (40 mg for 4 days is a typical dose). This will commence tumour kill, and the anti-inflammatory effect may be helpful to the proximal tubular injury caused by the excess light chains. In the MERIT study, Drayson and colleagues showed that single agent dexamethasone alone could have a profound impact in reducing FLC levels in the newly diagnosed MM patient with RI – outweighing any contribution that plasma exchange may have offered [10]. Addition of at least a second agent (ideally a triplet) is required within the initial 4 day period to increase the rate of tumour kill – it cannot be emphasised enough that the 'window of opportunity' to salvage kidney function and become independent of dialysis is a short one – possibly as little as 3 weeks, certainly 6 weeks. Clinical data shows that the reduction in FLC level at 21 days is highly predictive of the likelihood of renal recovery [2], and there is biopsy evidence of irreversible scarring by 6 weeks [1]. At present, there is a large body of evidence supporting the use of bortezomib as the second agent.

Bortezomib

Bortezomib is a dipeptide boronic acid analogue from the class of drugs known as proteasome inhibitors, blocking the degradation of nuclear factor kappa B inhibitor (NF-κBi) and thus the activation of NF-κB, removing an inhibitor of apoptosis. Once administered it undergoes oxidative hepatic metabolism [16]. First described in 1999, it was shown to be effective against myeloma cell lines in 2001 and rapidly entered clinical trials, achieving marketing authorisation in 2003. Early data examining bortezomib at reduced dose (1 mg/m^2) and standard doses (1.3 mg/m^2) showed a clinical benefit in 10 patients with relapsed/refractory myeloma (RRMM) and a creatinine clearance ≤30 mL/min [17]. Further data in 24 patients requiring dialysis who received variable doses of bortezomib alone or in combination demonstrated a response rate of 75%, thus demonstrating for this group of patients a therapeutic opportunity not previously seen commonly – a myeloma response and a renal response [18]. More recently it has been demonstrated that conventional doses (1.3 mg/m^2) are effective and tolerated in patients with low GFR or on dialysis [19].

Patients with multiple myeloma have excellent long-term outcomes after recovery from dialysis-dependent acute kidney injury. Newly diagnosed patients with severe RI are rarely a group included in large-scale studies. However, there are clues from such studies as to how this patient group can benefit. Dimopoulos analysed outcome based on renal function of patients treated within the VISTA study, where newly diagnosed patients were randomised between melphalan/prednisolone (MP) or bortezomib/melphalan/prednisolone (VMP) [20]. In the cohort with a GFR <50 mL/min, there was a higher rate of improvement in renal function to >60 mL/min (44% in the VMP arm vs 34% in the MP arm). Time to renal reversal was quicker in the VMP arm (2.1 months vs 2.4 months). Aside from the improvement that bortezomib offered, the authors suggest that melphalan may not be the best partner for bortezomib in the renally impaired as both arms had an elevated safety profile in this group of patients.

Perhaps the seminal paper in this group of patients is that by Ludwig and colleagues [21]. In a prospective study, they evaluated the activity of the combination of bortezomib, doxorubicin and dexamethasone in patients with AKI in the context of newly diagnosed or progressive previously treated disease. Patients were treated for up to 8 cycles. The initial dosing of 9 mg/m^2 doxorubicin on days 1, 4, 8 and 11 was reduced to days 1 and 4, with a reduction of bortezomib dose from 1.3 mg/m^2 on days 1, 4, 8 and 11 to 1.0 mg/m^2, following 2 deaths in a safety run-in. These doses were used for cycles 1–2 with the option to increase the dose if tolerated thereafter. There were 68 patients constituting the intention to treat cohort of which 58 were evaluable. The median number of cycles given was 8. The CR/nCR rate was 38% with 66% achieving PR or better. Thirty-one per cent of patients achieved renal CR, 7% renal PR and 24% renal MR – an overall renal response rate of 62%. Three out of nine dialysis-dependent patients became dialysis independent. The key finding was the link between myeloma response and renal response, with GFR increasing to a median of 59.6 mL/min in those achieving a CR/nCR/VGPR, 38.9 mL/min in those achieving a PR/MR and 16.8 mL/min in those with SD/PD. When the outcomes from the EuLITE study and others are added in [3, 13, 22], it is clear that a bortezomib-based triplet offers a significant myeloma and renal response combined.

Other Proteasome Inhibitors

Carfilzomib

Carfilzomib is an intravenous selective proteasome inhibitor with greater selectivity for the proteasome without inhibiting off-target proteases. Badros and colleagues treated 50 patients with varying degrees of RI (including some on dialysis) with escalating doses of carfilzomib up to 27 mg/m^2 per dose [23]. In this heavily pretreated group, an overall response rate (ORR) of 25.5% was seen. RI did not affect the likelihood of response. They confirmed that renal clearance is not a significant pathway for the elimination of carfilzomib (<1% of total dose recovered in urine samples within 24 hours post-dose).

The adverse effect (AE) profile was in line with those seen in other clinical trials using carfilzomib. There did not appear to be any clinically relevant nephrotoxicity. Thus there is unlikely to be a need to change schedule or dosing of carfilzomib in the treatment of myeloma patients with RI.

Ixazomib

Ixazomib is a selective, orally available, second-generation proteasome inhibitor administered as ixazomib citrate. Upon exposure to aqueous solutions or plasma, it rapidly hydrolyses to its active form ixazomib [24]. As with bortezomib and carfilzomib, it has been assessed in phase 1–3 studies in newly diagnosed and RR myeloma, demonstrating efficacy, particularly in combination with lenalidomide and dexamethasone [25]. Gupta and colleagues in a phase 1/1b study treated patients with normal renal function, severe RI (GFR <30 mL/min) and end-stage renal disease (ESRD) [26]. All patients received 3 mg of ixazomib on day 1 and, if tolerated, following a day 15 PK sample, could then proceed to receive 2.3 mg, 3 mg or 4 mg on days 1, 8 and 15 of a 28 day cycle. Dexamethasone could be used at the discretion of the investigator. PK showed that patients in the severe RI and ESRD groups had 38% and 39% higher systemic exposure to ixazomib, respectively, with a higher incidence of grade ≥3 treatment emergent AEs, serious AEs (SAEs) and discontinuations due to AEs. As a consequence, a reduced starting dose (3 mg) is recommended in these two patient groups. They were also able to demonstrate that ixazomib levels were not affected by HD.

Immunomodulatory Drugs

Thalidomide

Thalidomide is an immunomodulatory (IMiD) drug taken orally. It undergoes plasma hydrolysis and then hepatic metabolism generating active and non-active thalidomide metabolites. Thalidomide renal clearance is low (~1.15 mL/min), whereas whole body clearance is 170 mL/min, indicating renal function should have little impact on dosing [27]. There were early reports of fatal hyperkalaemia in patients with significant renal insufficiency who received thalidomide [28], but subsequently it has been used effectively in many patients. Despite being the first of the novel agents, there is surprisingly little prospective data on thalidomide in the renally impaired patient. The one significant study by Tosi et al. treated 31 patients with renal insufficiency (baseline clearance <50 mL/min), 7 of whom required haemodialysis [29]. They received 4 months of thalidomide (100 mg/day for 2 weeks escalated to 200 mg/day thereafter) with dexamethasone (40 mg/day days 1–4, 9–12 and 17–20 on odd cycles and days 1–4 on even cycles). Patients then underwent stem cell mobilisation with a view to autologous stem cell transplant (ASCT). Seventy-four per cent of patients achieved a PR or better in response to induction. Fifty-five per cent of patients improved renal function to a level >50 mL/min – as seen with bortezomib, renal response was linked to myeloma response. The toxicity profile was similar to that seen in patients with normal renal function. Deep vein thrombosis was seen in three patients.

Thalidomide combined with the alkylator bendamustine and dexamethasone (BTD) has activity in relapsed myeloma [30]. Bendamustine can be used in RI [31, 32], so the BTD triplet is a treatment option in such patients requiring therapy.

Thrombosis can be a significant issue in myeloma patients with RI treated with thalidomide and other IMiDs. The placement of a tunnelled line for the purpose of HD is a risk factor as is the presence of an active cancer. Initiation of therapy with thalidomide (or other immunomodulatory drugs) along with dexamethasone significantly increases the risk of thrombosis further. Therefore thought has to be given about risk reduction in this patient group. The author's own practice is to use low molecular weight heparin dose adjusted according to anti-Xa levels. Thrombosis of a dialysis catheter (or a fistula fashioned for long-term HD) can cause significant problems in the management of patients otherwise and is thus best avoided.

Lenalidomide

Lenalidomide is a thalidomide analogue, taken orally. PK evaluation shows a clear relationship between renal function and handling of lenalidomide with total clearance decreasing drastically as renal function lessens [33]. Dialysis does remove lenalidomide, so the dosing adjustments in the renally impaired need to take account of the degree of RI – with correction of dose upward if the patient ends up requiring dialysis.

There is prospective data available on the use of lenalidomide in renally impaired patients – some specifically planned and others post-trial subgroup analyses. Ludwig and colleagues prospectively evaluated the activity and tolerance of lenalidomide and dexamethasone in 35 patients with AKI secondary to myeloma [34]. The dose of lenalidomide was adjusted according to the degree of RI. High-dose dexamethasone was used in cycle 1 and de-escalated subsequently. The myeloma response rate (PR or greater) was 68.6% with a renal response rate of 45.7% – the median eGFR improving from 17.1 mL/min to 39.1 mL/min. Haematological toxicity and infections were amongst the commonest toxicities – and whilst these are seen in myeloma patients with normal renal function treated with lenalidomide, it is clear that dose adjustment is required frequently in patients with RI to help manage the toxicities seen.

The Frontline Investigation of Revlimid plus Dexamethasone vs Standard Thalidomide (FIRST) trial compared lenalidomide and dexamethasone (Rd) continuous until PD vs 18 months Rd vs 10 months melphalan, prednisolone and thalidomide (MPT) [35]. Within this study, lenalidomide dosing could be adapted according to the patient's renal function at the time. 1623 patients were randomised within the study of which 24% had normal renal function, 44.1%

had mild RI, 22.9% had moderate RI and 9.1% had severe RI (but not requiring dialysis). The trial as a whole showed a significant benefit for continuous Rd for PFS, RFS and OS. However, in patients with severe RI, there was no clear PFS benefit for continuous Rd – indeed there was a shorter PFS across all three arms in this subgroup. There was no difference in overall response rate in this subgroup (nor in the patients with no RI), but patients with severe RI had lower response rates compared to the other renal subgroups. Improved renal function was generally seen across all subgroups with a trend for Rd to give a higher chance of improvement. Patients with severe RI had the shortest median duration of treatment (6.8 months) compared to 18.9 months for the other renal subgroups. In all treatment arms, the incidence of anaemia increased with severity of RI. So whilst the trial had not been specifically designed to examine the treatment of patients with severe RI, the generous inclusion criteria mean that we have learnt a lot about the use of lenalidomide in this patient group [36].

Pomalidomide

Pomalidomide is the third IMiD to achieve marketing authorisation for the treatment of relapsed myeloma. Data is available on effectiveness and tolerability in patients with RI. In the MM-013 study, three cohorts (moderate RI eGFR 30 to <45 mL/min, severe RI eGFR<30 mL/min and severe RI requiring HD) were treated with pomalidomide plus low-dose dexamethasone [37]. In total, 81 patients were recruited to the study. ORRs were 39.4%, 32.4% and 14.3% across the 3 cohorts, respectively, with 100%, 79.4% and 78.6% achieving disease control. Median overall survival was 16.4 months, 11.8 months and 5.2 months, respectively. No patients in the latter cohort became independent of HD. So in this study, it can be seen that whilst pomalidomide and dexamethasone is deliverable in patients with severe RI, we can also see some other learning points. Patients who are dialysis-dependent with late-stage myeloma tend not to do as well as those patients who have remained independent of dialysis – and this may reflect both disease biology but also the fact that dialysis dependence is in itself a burdensome co-morbidity. In a pooled analysis of three clinical trials of pomalidomide and low-dose dexamethasone (MM-002, MM-003 and MM-010), Siegel and colleagues showed that patients with moderate RI (creatinine clearance ≥30 mL/min to ≤60 mL/min) had a similar response ORR, PFS, TTP and DOR compared to patients with no RI, but overall survival was shorter (10.5 months vs 14.0 months, $p = 0.004$), supporting the idea that RI in late-stage myeloma has a negative impact on survival [38].

HDAC Inhibitors

Panobinostat (previously LBH589) is a hydroxamic acid-derived histone deacetylase (HDAC) inhibitor shown to have significant anti-myeloma activity as a single agent and in combination with bortezomib and lenalidomide in vitro [39]. It is licensed to be used in conjunction with bortezomib and dexamethasone. The PANORAMA 1 trial showed a significant PFS benefit of panobinostat with bortezomib and dexamethasone versus a control arm of bortezomib and dexamethasone. However, there were significant AEs – particularly GI toxicity. These do seem to be reduced by changing bortezomib to a once weekly schedule [40]. There is very little data on the use of panobinostat in patients with RI. PK studies indicate no change in systemic exposure with increasing severity of renal impairment [41]. A very small case series describes the use of panobinostat in combination with bortezomib and dexamethasone in three patients requiring HD [42]. In all three cases, there was a myeloma response seen, but for two cases, continuation of therapy was not possible due to tolerability, and in the third patient, treatment was discontinued at the patient's request. At present therefore, there is no data set to inform treatment in this patient group, and thus if the triplet is used, careful clinical evaluation before and during therapy is required with consideration of dose modification of bortezomib and/or panobinostat if AEs occur.

Monoclonal Antibodies

Daratumumab is a monoclonal antibody that targets CD38, preferentially expressed on the surface of myeloma cells. It is licensed as a single agent and also in combination, with lenalidomide and dexamethasone (DRd) [43] and with bortezomib and dexamethasone (DVd) [44] for the treatment of relapsed myeloma and in combination with bortezomib, melphalan and prednisolone (DVMP) [45] and bortezomib, thalidomide and dexamethasone (DVTd) [46] for the newly diagnosed patient. Daratumumab combinations offer remarkable response rates and duration of response, linked to high rates of minimal residual disease (MRD) negativity. Daratumumab is not metabolised in the kidney. Originally given as an intravenous infusion it is now available as a subcutaneous formulation. The volume of infusion and the rate of infusion of the intravenous preparation can potentially be a challenge to patients with severe RI, but careful management in liaison with renal physicians can help negate the risk in the few patients requring intravenous treatment. There is an ongoing phase 2 study evaluating daratumumab single agent in patients with RI (ichgcp.net/clinical-trials-registry/NCT03450057). The ALCYONE study reported on DVMP vs VMP. Cavo et al. reported on the impact of baseline renal function of the efficacy and safety within the ALCYONE study (meeting abstract) [47]. 295 out of 706 patients had a baseline creatinine clearance (CrCl) of ≥40 ml/min to ≤60 mL/min. The benefit for ORR and PFS seen for the DVMP arm as a whole was also seen in those with RI with no increase in infusion reactions. There is therefore some evidence available to justify confidence in using daratumumab in RI.

Elotuzumab is a monoclonal antibody targeting cell surface signalling lymphocytic activation molecule family member 7 (SLAM-F7) and is licensed in the USA when used in combination with lenalidomide and dexamethasone (Elo-Rd) [48] and also with pomalidomide and dexamethasone for the treatment of relapsed myeloma (Elo-Pd) [49]. In a phase 1b study, Elo-Rd was given to patients with normal renal function, severe RI (CrCl<30 mL/min not requiring HD) and ESRD requiring HD [50]. The mean elotuzumab concentrations were comparable across all groups, and there were no differences in maximum observed serum concentration or area under the concentration-time curve. The findings support the use of elotuzumab in severe RI without dose adjustment.

Autologous Stem Cell Transplantation

For younger fitter patients, high-dose melphalan and stem cell rescue (autologous stem cell transplant – ASCT) remain the standard of care to consolidate the gains made by induction therapy more than 20 years after the first trial showing benefit in terms of PFS and OS [51]. Whilst the concept remains under challenge, even the most contemporary trial reporting presently shows a benefit for ASCT [52]. Patients with significant RI have been excluded from randomised transplant trials, but there is a wealth of observational and small-scale prospective single arm studies that help us to understand how patients with RI can be offered and undergo ASCT for clinical benefit. Because of the inter-patient variation in melphalan pharmacokinetics, there is inconsistent data and advice on whether a reduction in melphalan dosage is required for patients with RI. When CrCl is <50 mL/min, then a reduction from the standard melphalan dose of 200 mg/m^2 to 140 mg/m^2 is often applied. There is conflicting evidence if this has an impact on outcome, with a recent report suggesting not [53]. However, a large retrospective registry study comparing melphalan dose across varying degrees of RI showed that for moderate RI (CrCl 30-59 mL/min), melphalan dose reduction compromised 5-year PFS

(18% for 140 mg/m^2 vs 46% for 200 mg/m^2 $p = 0.009$). In severe RI (CrCl<30 mL/min), there was no significant difference in 5-year PFS [54]. What is clear when there is no dose reduction applied for RI is that toxicity is more significant, particularly mucositis, GI toxicity and infection [55]. For patients who are HD-dependent, initial reports of ASCT indicated high rates of mortality. As supportive care and patient selection has improved, it has become a therapy that can be offered with little excess risk [56, 57]. Certainly now, RI of itself cannot be seen as a barrier to ASCT.

Considerations for the Future

The current approach to the management of renal impairment in myeloma – particularly acute kidney injury requiring renal replacement therapy – is heavily focussed on the reduction of circulating FLCs, thereby reducing the rate at which ongoing injury occurs, buying time for renal recovery to commence. However, there has been limited focus on two other aspects of the acute kidney injury which might present a complementary approach to further improve outcomes beyond what has been seen over the last decade.

Proximal Tubule Injury as a Potential Therapeutic Target

It is now quite clear that when there is excess circulating free light chain sufficient to pass through the glomerulus and saturate the proximal tubule 'recycling' mechanism, an inflammatory environment develops due to activation of STAT1 [58]. As a consequence, IL-1β (pro-inflammatory) and TGF-β (pro-fibrotic) are produced, ultimately causing the fibrotic proximal tubulopathy that is one of the hallmarks of myeloma kidney. There is experimental evidence that this process might be addressed by ruxolitinib, a JAK-2 inhibitor more commonly used to treat myelofibrosis. This would appear to be an area suitable for exploration within a clinical trial.

Free Light Chain-Uromodulin Interaction as a Potential Therapeutic Target

The classic cast nephropathy injury is the intraluminal deposition of waxy casts. These casts are formed by precipitation after the binding of light chain within duct fluid with uromodulin (Tamm-Horsfall protein). It would thus be logical to try and block this interaction, allowing light chain to pass through freely. There is interesting animal model data to suggest that this could be a potential route to future therapy [59].

Summary

Renal impairment in myeloma is a common event. Severe RI presenting acutely requiring dialysis should be considered a medical emergency. Prompt evaluation and institution of corrective measures can improve the clinical condition of the patient – and indeed help avoid dialysis. The commencement of anti-myeloma therapy is a high priority to improve the chances of reduction in the level of circulating FLC, thus reducing the ongoing rate of cast nephropathy. Reduction in FLC level by day 21 [2] is strongly predictive of eventual outcome. There is a short 6-week period to effect reversal of the renal injury [1], so consideration should be given to changing therapy based on the day 21 FLC value if there has been little response.

There is no data that currently supports the use of mechanical removal of light chains. Certainly, plasma exchange has no role. High cut-off dialysis membranes remain unproven and should only be used in the context of a clinical trial.

Chemotherapy options in the patient with RI are now essentially the same as any other myeloma patient. For some drugs, care should be taken in dosing. Triplets should be considered the standard of care as any other patient group. For younger, fitter patients, autologous stem cell transplantation should be considered as part of their standard of care. As a consequence of clinicians having better treatments at their disposal, the outcome for patients with RI has improved at a faster rate than other patient subgroups [60]. However, there is a significant unmet need in this patient group – therapies that target the renal injury and the interaction between free light chains and uromodulin are required to treat the renal problem 'at source'.

References

1. Basnayake K, Cheung CK, Sheaff M, et al. Differential progression of renal scarring and determinants of late renal recovery in sustained dialysis dependent acute kidney injury secondary to myeloma kidney. J Clin Pathol. 2010;63:884–7.
2. Hutchison CA, Cockwell P, Stringer S, et al. Early reduction of serum-free light chains associates with renal recovery in myeloma kidney. J Am Soc Nephrol. 2011;22:1129–36.
3. Dimopoulos MA, Roussou M, Gavriatopoulou M, et al. Outcomes of newly diagnosed myeloma patients requiring dialysis: renal recovery, importance of rapid response and survival benefit. Blood Cancer J. 2017;7:e571.
4. Sanders PW, Booker BB. Pathobiology of cast nephropathy from human Bence Jones proteins. J Clin Invest. 1992;89:630–9.
5. (1984) Analysis and management of renal failure in fourth MRC myelomatosis trial. MRC working party on leukaemia in adults. Br Med J (Clin Res Ed) 288:1411–1416.
6. Johnson WJ, Kyle RA, Pineda AA, O'Brien PC, Holley KE. Treatment of renal failure associated with multiple myeloma. Plasmapheresis, hemodialysis, and chemotherapy. Arch Intern Med. 1990;150:863–9.
7. Zucchelli P, Pasquali S, Cagnoli L, Ferrari G. Controlled plasma exchange trial in acute renal failure due to multiple myeloma. Kidney Int. 1988;33:1175–80.
8. Moist L, Nesrallah G, Kortas C, Espirtu E, Ostbye T, Clark WF. Plasma exchange in rapidly progressive renal failure due to

multiple myeloma. A retrospective case series. Am J Nephrol. 1999;19:45–50.

9. Clark WF, Stewart AK, Rock GA, Sternbach M, Sutton DM, Barrett BJ, Heidenheim AP, Garg AX, Churchill DN, and the Canadian Apheresis Group. Plasma exchange when myeloma presents as acute renal failure: a randomized, controlled trial. Ann Intern Med. 2005;143:777.
10. Drayson MT, Behrens J, Cohen D, Iggo N, Bell SE, Jackson G, Gregory W, Gaskin J. In patients with myeloma and renal failure free light chain levels (SFLC) can be reduced greatly within 2 weeks and lower SFLC levels are associated with a better chance of renal recovery. Haematologica. 2012;97:355.
11. Hutchison CA, Cockwell P, Reid S, et al. Efficient removal of immunoglobulin free light chains by hemodialysis for multiple myeloma: in vitro and in vivo studies. J Am Soc Nephrol. 2007;18:886–95.
12. Bridoux F, Carron P-L, Pegourie B, et al. Effect of high-cutoff hemodialysis vs conventional hemodialysis on hemodialysis Independence among patients with myeloma cast nephropathy: a randomized clinical trial. JAMA. 2017;318:2099–110.
13. Hutchison CA, Cockwell P, Moroz V, et al. High cutoff versus high-flux haemodialysis for myeloma cast nephropathy in patients receiving bortezomib-based chemotherapy (EuLITE): a phase 2 randomised controlled trial. Lancet Haematol. 2019;6:e217–28.
14. Barlogie B, Smith L, Alexanian R. Effective treatment of advanced multiple myeloma refractory to alkylating agents. N Engl J Med. 1984;310:1353–6.
15. Alexanian R, Dimopoulos MA, Delasalle K, Barlogie B. Primary dexamethasone treatment of multiple myeloma. Blood. 1992;80:887–90.
16. Pekol T, Daniels JS, Labutti J, Parsons I, Nix D, Baronas E, Hsieh F, Gan L-S, Miwa G. Human metabolism of the proteasome inhibitor bortezomib: identification of circulating metabolites. Drug Metab Dispos. 2005;33:771–7.
17. Jagannath S, Barlogie B, Berenson JR, et al. Bortezomib in recurrent and/or refractory multiple myeloma. Initial clinical experience in patients with impared renal function. Cancer. 2005;103:1195–200.
18. Chanan-Khan AA, Kaufman JL, Mehta J, Richardson PG, Miller KC, Lonial S, Munshi NC, Schlossman R, Tariman J, Singhal S. Activity and safety of bortezomib in multiple myeloma

patients with advanced renal failure: a multicenter retrospective study. Blood. 2007;109:2604–6.
19. Leal TB, Remick SC, Takimoto CH, et al. Dose-escalating and pharmacological study of bortezomib in adult cancer patients with impaired renal function: a National Cancer Institute Organ Dysfunction Working Group Study. Cancer Chemother Pharmacol. 2011;68:1439–47.
20. Dimopoulos MA, Richardson PG, Schlag R, et al. VMP (Bortezomib, Melphalan, and Prednisone) is active and well tolerated in newly diagnosed patients with multiple myeloma with moderately impaired renal function, and results in reversal of renal impairment: cohort analysis of the phase III VISTA study. J Clin Oncol. 2009;27:6086–93.
21. Ludwig H, Adam Z, Hajek R, et al. Light chain-induced acute renal failure can be reversed by bortezomib-doxorubicin-dexamethasone in multiple myeloma: results of a phase II study. J Clin Oncol. 2010;28:4635–41.
22. Dimopoulos MA, Roussou M, Gavriatopoulou M, et al. Bortezomib-based triplets are associated with a high probability of dialysis independence and rapid renal recovery in newly diagnosed myeloma patients with severe renal failure or those requiring dialysis. Am J Hematol. 2016;91:499–502.
23. Badros AZ, Vij R, Martin T, Zonder JA, Kunkel L, Wang Z, Lee S, Wong AF, Niesvizky R. Carfilzomib in multiple myeloma patients with renal impairment: pharmacokinetics and safety. Leukemia. 2013;27:1707–14.
24. Kumar SK, Bensinger WI, Zimmerman TM, et al. Phase 1 study of weekly dosing with the investigational oral proteasome inhibitor ixazomib in relapsed/refractory multiple myeloma. Blood. 2014;124:1047–55.
25. Kumar SK, Berdeja JG, Niesvizky R, et al. Ixazomib, lenalidomide, and dexamethasone in patients with newly diagnosed multiple myeloma: long-term follow-up including ixazomib maintenance. Leukemia. 2019;33:1736–46.
26. Gupta N, Hanley MJ, Harvey RD, et al. A pharmacokinetics and safety phase 1/1b study of oral ixazomib in patients with multiple myeloma and severe renal impairment or end-stage renal disease requiring haemodialysis. Br J Haematol. 2016;174:748–59.
27. Izzedine H, Launay-Vacher V, Deray G. Thalidomide for the nephrologist. Nephrol Dial Transplant. 2005;20:2011–2.
28. Harris E, Behrens J, Samson D, Rahemtulla A, Russell NH, Byrne JL. Use of thalidomide in patients with myeloma and

renal failure may be associated with unexplained hyperkalaemia. Br J Haematol. 2003;122:160–1.
29. Tosi P, Zamagni E, Tacchetti P, et al. Thalidomide-dexamethasone as induction therapy before autologous stem cell transplantation in patients with newly diagnosed multiple myeloma and renal insufficiency. Biol Blood Marrow Transplant. 2010;16:1115–21.
30. Schey S, Brown SR, Tillotson A-L, et al. Bendamustine, thalidomide and dexamethasone combination therapy for relapsed/refractory myeloma patients: results of the MUKone randomized dose selection trial. Br J Haematol. 2015;170:336–48.
31. Ettleson M, Bongers KS, Vitale K, Perissinotti AJ, Phillips T, Marini BL. Successful use of cytarabine and bendamustine in a patient with mantle cell lymphoma and acute renal failure using intermittent hemodialysis: a case report. J Oncol Pharm Pract. 2019;25:731–4.
32. Pönisch W, Holzvogt B, Plötze M, et al. Bendamustine and prednisone in combination with bortezomib (BPV) in the treatment of patients with newly diagnosed/untreated multiple myeloma. J Cancer Res Clin Oncol. 2014;140:1947–56.
33. Chen N, Lau H, Kong L, Kumar G, Zeldis JB, Knight R, Laskin OL. Pharmacokinetics of lenalidomide in subjects with various degrees of renal impairment and in subjects on hemodialysis. J Clin Pharmacol. 2007;47:1466–75.
34. Ludwig H, Rauch E, Kuehr T, et al. Lenalidomide and dexamethasone for acute light chain-induced renal failure: a phase II study. Haematologica. 2015;100:385–91.
35. Facon T, Dimopoulos MA, Dispenzieri A, et al. Final analysis of survival outcomes in the phase 3 FIRST trial of up-front treatment for multiple myeloma. Blood. 2018;131:301–10.
36. Dimopoulos MA, Cheung MC, Roussel M, et al. Impact of renal impairment on outcomes with lenalidomide and dexamethasone treatment in the FIRST trial, a randomized, open-label phase 3 trial in transplant-ineligible patients with multiple myeloma. Haematologica. 2016;101:363–70.
37. Weisel KC, Dimopoulos MA, Moreau P, et al. Analysis of renal impairment in MM-003, a phase III study of pomalidomide + low – dose dexamethasone versus high – dose dexamethasone in refractory or relapsed and refractory multiple myeloma. Haematologica. 2016;101:872–8.
38. Siegel DS, Weisel KC, Dimopoulos MA, et al. Pomalidomide plus low-dose dexamethasone in patients with relapsed/refractory

multiple myeloma and moderate renal impairment: a pooled analysis of three clinical trials. Leuk Lymphoma. 2016;57:2833–8.
39. Maiso P, Carvajal-Vergara X, Ocio EM, López-Pérez R, Mateo G, Gutiérrez N, Atadja P, Pandiella A, Miguel JFS. The histone deacetylase inhibitor LBH589 is a potent antimyeloma agent that overcomes drug resistance. Cancer Res. 2006;66:5781–9.
40. San-Miguel JF, Hungria VTM, Yoon S-S, et al. Panobinostat plus bortezomib and dexamethasone: impact of dose intensity and administration frequency on safety in the PANORAMA 1 trial. Br J Haematol. 2017;179:66–74.
41. Sharma S, Witteveen PO, Lolkema MP, Hess D, Gelderblom H, Hussain SA, Porro MG, Waldron E, Valera S-Z, Mu S. A phase I, open-label, multicenter study to evaluate the pharmacokinetics and safety of oral panobinostat in patients with advanced solid tumors and varying degrees of renal function. Cancer Chemother Pharmacol. 2015;75:87–95.
42. Sekiguchi Y, Takizawa H, Inano T, et al. Three cases of relapsed/refractory multiple myeloma under hemodialysis treated with panobinostat/bortezomib/dexamethasone (FVD). Int J Hematol. 2017;106:581–7.
43. Dimopoulos MA, Oriol A, Nahi H, et al. Daratumumab, lenalidomide, and dexamethasone for multiple myeloma. N Engl J Med. 2016;375:1319–31.
44. Palumbo A, Chanan-Khan A, Weisel K, et al. Daratumumab, bortezomib, and dexamethasone for multiple myeloma. N Engl J Med. 2016;375:754–66.
45. Mateos M-V, Dimopoulos MA, Cavo M, et al. Daratumumab plus bortezomib, melphalan, and prednisone for untreated myeloma. N Engl J Med. 2018;378:518–28.
46. Moreau P, Attal M, Hulin C, et al. Bortezomib, thalidomide, and dexamethasone with or without daratumumab before and after autologous stem-cell transplantation for newly diagnosed multiple myeloma (CASSIOPEIA): a randomised, open-label, phase 3 study. Lancet. 2019;394:29–38.
47. Cavo M, Dimopoulos MA, San-Miguel J, et al. Impact of baseline renal function on efficacy and safety of daratumumab plus bortezomib-melphalan-prednisone (VMP) in patients (Pts) with newly diagnosed multiple myeloma (NDMM) ineligible for transplantation (ALCYONE). JCO. 2018;36:e20024.
48. Lonial S, Dimopoulos M, Palumbo A, et al. Elotuzumab therapy for relapsed or refractory multiple myeloma. N Engl J Med. 2015;373:621–31.

49. Dimopoulos MA, Dytfeld D, Grosicki S, et al. Elotuzumab plus pomalidomide and dexamethasone for multiple myeloma. N Engl J Med. 2018;379:1811–22.
50. Berdeja J, Jagannath S, Zonder J, et al. Pharmacokinetics and safety of elotuzumab combined with lenalidomide and dexamethasone in patients with multiple myeloma and various levels of renal impairment: results of a phase Ib study. Clin Lymphoma Myeloma Leuk. 2016;16:129–38.
51. Attal M, Harousseau JL, Stoppa AM, et al. A prospective, randomized trial of autologous bone marrow transplantation and chemotherapy in multiple myeloma. Intergroupe Français du Myélome. N Engl J Med. 1996;335:91–7.
52. Attal M, Lauwers-Cances V, Hulin C, et al. Lenalidomide, bortezomib, and dexamethasone with transplantation for myeloma. N Engl J Med. 2017;376:1311–20.
53. Augeul-Meunier K, Chretien M-L, Stoppa A-M, et al. Extending autologous transplantation as first line therapy in multiple myeloma patients with severe renal impairment: a retrospective study by the SFGM-TC. Bone Marrow Transplant. 2018;53:749–55.
54. Mahindra A, Hari P, Fraser R, et al. Autologous hematopoietic cell transplantation for multiple myeloma patients with renal insufficiency: a center for international blood and marrow transplant research analysis. Bone Marrow Transplant. 2017;52:1616–22.
55. Sweiss K, Patel S, Culos K, Oh A, Rondelli D, Patel P. Melphalan 200 mg/m2 in patients with renal impairment is associated with increased short-term toxicity but improved response and longer treatment-free survival. Bone Marrow Transplant. 2016;51:1337–41.
56. El Fakih R, Fox P, Popat U, et al. Autologous hematopoietic stem cell transplantation in dialysis-dependent myeloma patients. Clin Lymphoma Myeloma Leuk. 2015;15:472–6.
57. Lee C-K, Zangari M, Barlogie B, et al. Dialysis-dependent renal failure in patients with myeloma can be reversed by high-dose myeloablative therapy and autotransplant. Bone Marrow Transplant. 2004;33:823–8.
58. Ying W-Z, Li X, Rangarajan S, Feng W, Curtis LM, Sanders PW. Immunoglobulin light chains generate proinflammatory and profibrotic kidney injury. J Clin Invest. 2019;130:2792–806.

59. Ying W-Z, Allen CE, Curtis LM, Aaron KJ, Sanders PW. Mechanism and prevention of acute kidney injury from cast nephropathy in a rodent model. J Clin Invest. 2012;122:1777–85.
60. Evison F, Sangha J, Yadav P, Aung YS, Sharif A, Pinney JA, Drayson MT, Cook M, Cockwell P. A population-based study of the impact of dialysis on mortality in multiple myeloma. Br J Haematol. 2018;180:588–91.
61. Hendrayana T, Wilmer A, Kurth V, Schmidt-Wolf IG, Jaehde U. Anticancer dose adjustment for patients with renal and hepatic dysfunction: from scientific evidence to clinical application. Sci Pharm. 2017;85(1):8. https://doi.org/10.3390/scipharm85010008.
62. Revlimid 25 mg Hard Capsules – Summary of Product Characteristics (SmPC) – (emc). https://www.medicines.org.uk/emc/product/10047/smpc. Accessed 31 Oct 2019.

Correction to: The Pathophysiology of Myeloma Bone Disease: Bone Remodelling and the Role of Osteoclasts

Rebecca E. Andrews, Andrew D. Chantry, and A. John Ashcroft

Correction to:
Chapter 2 in: E. Zamagni (ed.), Management of Bone Disease and Kidney Failure in Multiple Myeloma, https://doi.org/10.1007/978-3-030-63662-3_2

The book was inadvertently published with the captions of all the figures within text. The correct presentation is given here.

The updated version of this chapter can be found at https://doi.org/10.1007/978-3-030-63662-3_2

E. Zamagni (ed.), *Management of Bone Disease and Kidney Failure in Multiple Myeloma*,
https://doi.org/10.1007/978-3-030-63662-3_11

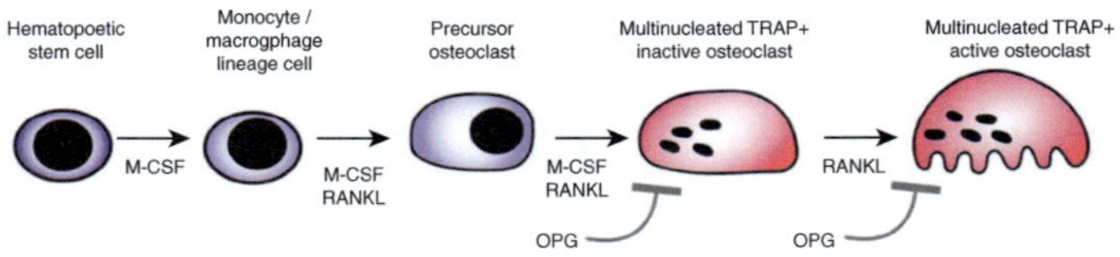

Figure 2.1 Osteoclastogenesis. Osteoclasts are derived from hematopoietic stem cells. In the presence of factors such as macrophage colony-stimulating factor (M-CSF) and receptor activator of nuclear factor kappa B ligand (RANKL), precursor OC cells differentiate into multinucleated osteoclast cells, which when activated are capable of bone resorption. Osteoclastogenesis can be inhibited by the production of OPG, which can bind to RANKL, preventing it binding to RANK on the OC cell surface

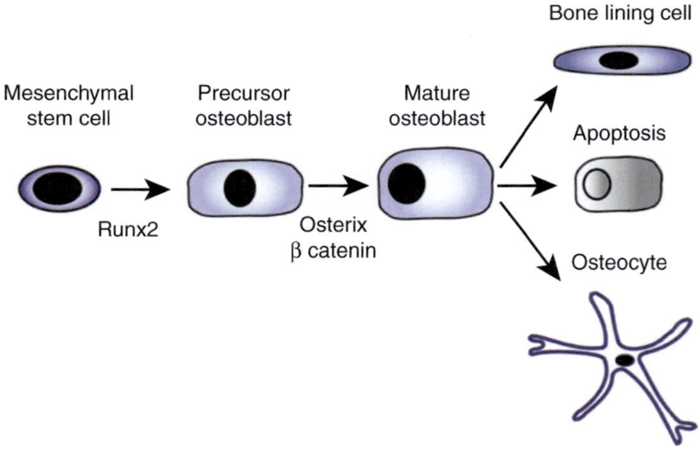

Figure 2.2 Osteoblast differentiation. Osteoblasts are derived from mesenchymal stem cells. Commitment to the osteoblast lineage is regulated by multiple pathways, of which the more established involve Wnt signalling cascades. Mature osteoblasts subsequently either apoptose, become entrapped within the bone matrix to form osteocytes or differentiate into bone-lining cells

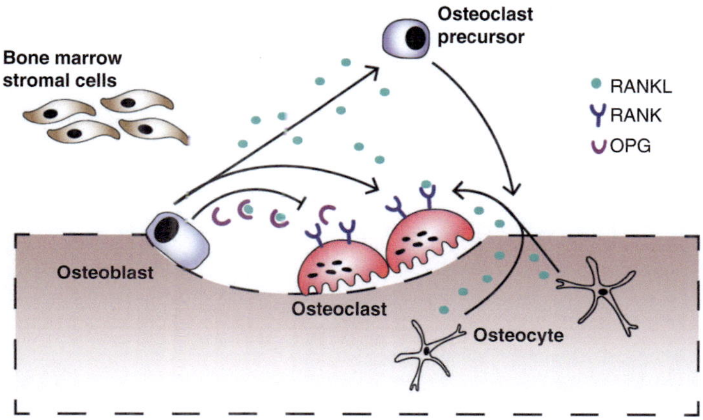

FIGURE 2.3 RANKL/RANK/OPG interaction. There is a close relationship between RANKL and OPG to either drive or antagonise OC differentiation, function and survival. RANKL is produced by both osteocytes and osteoblasts, and when bound to RANK on the surface of osteoclast precursors and immature osteoclasts, differentiation and maturation take place. This signalling pathway is moderated by osteoprotegerin (OPG), a decoy receptor to RANKL which is expressed by osteoblasts, to downregulate OC formation

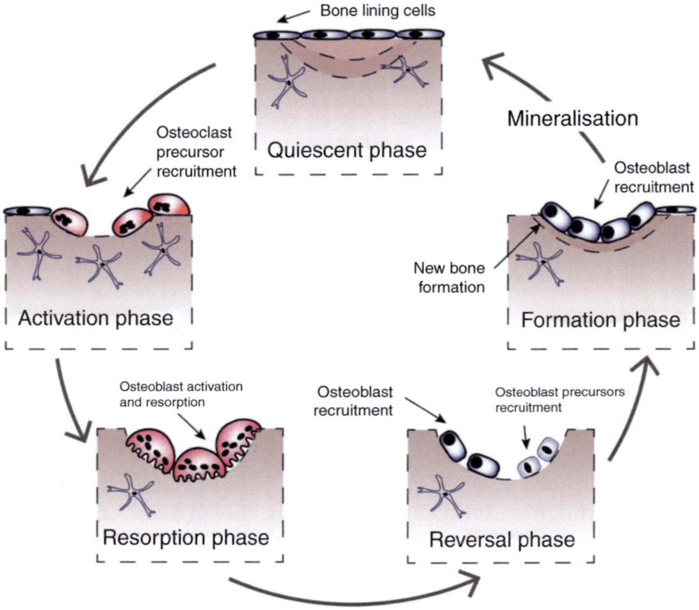

FIGURE 2.4 Physiological bone remodelling. Bone remodelling involves five distinct phases. Initially, bone microdamage or mechanical loading is recognised by osteocyte cells. Osteocyte-mediated intracellular signalling then triggers an activation phase in which osteoclast precursor cells are recruited to the area of the bone. Subsequent osteoclast maturation, recruitment and bone resorption follow. It is not understood what leads to the transition from resorption to formation, but in this so-called reversal phase, the osteoclasts' role is complete, and osteoblast precursors are recruited. The final active phase is that of bone formation. Osteoblasts lay down osteoid (a new collagen matrix) which will be later mineralised. On completion of the cycle, osteoblast cells either apoptose, become engulfed in the matrix and become osteocytes, or differentiate into bone lining cells that protect the surface of the new bone

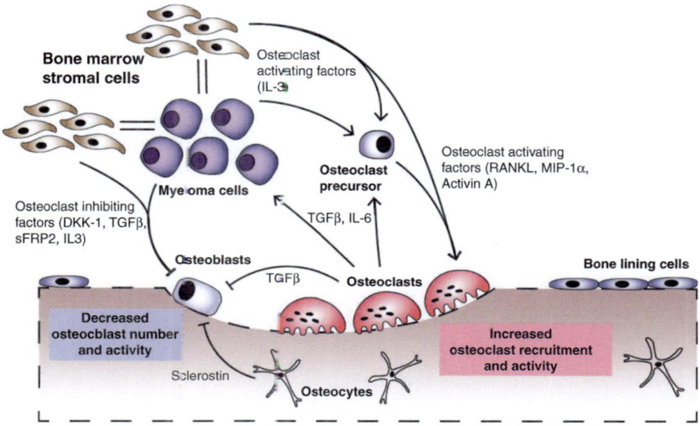

FIGURE 2.5 Myeloma bone disease: a vicious cycle. The pathophysiology of myeloma bone disease: Cellular interaction between myeloma plasma cells (MPCs) and bone marrow stromal cells (BMSCs) leads to factors that influence the equilibrium of bone turnover. Osteoclast-activating factors (e.g. IL-3, RANKL, MIP-1α and activin A) are released both from myeloma cells directly and indirect upregulation as a result of adhesion between MPCs and BMSCs. Increased resorption results in increased release of factors such as TGFβ and IL-6 from the bone marrow matrix. These promote a positive feedback with upregulation of MPC and osteoclast precursor proliferation, as well as inhibiting osteoblastogenesis. Osteoblast-inhibiting factors (e.g. DKK-1, TGFβ, sFRP2, IL-3) are also released as a result of the presence of MPCs and their interaction with BMSCs. These factors antagonise osteoblast differentiation and function. Sclerostin released from osteocytes is also upregulated in the presence of MPCs, which also inhibits osteoblast function. The overall effect of this is an increase in osteoclast activity and decreased osteoblast activity, resulting in osteolytic bone disease

Index

E. Zamagni (ed.), *Management of Bone Disease and Kidney Failure in Multiple Myeloma*,
https://doi.org/10.1007/978-3-030-63662-3

MIX
Papier aus verantwortungsvollen Quellen
Paper from responsible sources
FSC® C105338

If you have any concerns about our products,
you can contact us on
ProductSafety@springernature.com

In case Publisher is established outside the EU,
the EU authorized representative is:
Springer Nature Customer Service Center GmbH
Europaplatz 3, 69115 Heidelberg, Germany

Printed by Libri Plureos GmbH
in Hamburg, Germany